THE GAME OF MY LIFE

THE GAME OF MY LIFE

GARY ABLETT
MY AUTOBIOGRAPHY

Sport Media

To Jacqueline, Scarlet, Reece, Riley,
Josh and Fraser

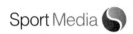

Copyright text: Gary Ablett.
Gary Ablett has asserted his right under the Copyright, Designs
and Patents Act 1988 to be identified as the author of this work.

A CIP catalogue record for this book
is available from the British Library.

Published in Great Britain in hardback form in 2012.
Published and produced by: Trinity Mirror Sport Media,
PO Box 48, Old Hall Street, Liverpool L69 3EB.

ISBN: 9781906802844

Photographs/images: Liverpool Daily Post & Echo,
Press Association Images, Mirrorpix, Getty Images,
Everton Former Players Foundation, Gary Ablett collection.
With thanks to Darren Griffiths at Everton Football Club
and Stephen Done at Liverpool Football Club.
Every effort has been made to obtain the necessary permissions with
reference to illustrative copyright material.
Any oversight will be rectified at the earliest available opportunity.

Printed and bound by CPI Group (UK) Ltd, Croydon, CR0 4YY

Contents

Introduction

This Is Gary's Story

It was December 23, 2011, when a text message came through to my mobile phone: "I'm okay mate. Hope you're fine. Cover pretty good. See you soon, Gary."

They were just a few short sentences, a brief thumbs up to the proposed jacket design for the autobiography on which we had been working, but they were enough to put my mind at rest. I'd not heard from Gary for a couple of weeks before that and had started to worry that he had taken a turn for the worse in his fight against cancer.

Of course, I realised that non-Hodgkin's lymphoma was a serious, life-threatening illness, but having seen him virtually every week for the previous six months I also knew that Gary Ablett was a fighter. Someone who had fought to overcome the odds throughout the course of his playing career and who had represented, in his own words, "two of the biggest clubs in the world."

Whatever the doctors might have said to him, I still hoped – and genuinely believed – he would not be beaten. He would pull through.

The text message was the last time I heard from Gary.

Christmas came and went and I was looking forward to seeing him again in the new year when I received a phone call on January 2 from another journalist saying he had passed away. It came as a terrible shock. Desperately sad.

Gary didn't remember, but the first time I met him was in the locker room at Portal Golf Club, near Tarporley, the morning after Everton had been knocked out of the European Cup Winners' Cup by Feyenoord back in 1995. Joe Royle's players were taking part in a golf day and, as the reporter starting out on The Evertonian magazine, I went along to get some interviews in the bag. Gary was one of the players who gave me 20 minutes of his time, happy to answer my list of questions, and I left with a notebook full of interviews.

In the years that followed, I spoke with him again while he was coaching Liverpool's reserve team, but it wasn't until the summer of 2011 that I really got to know him. Having fallen ill, and having been forced to take time out of coaching, Gary was apparently interested in writing a book about his life.

Straight away it struck me that his story was different to that of other footballers. He'd had a good career, and one that stood up to scrutiny, but his battle for health broadened the tale's appeal and he was eager to offer a positive message to anyone else who was suffering from the disease.

Colin Wood, the esteemed former Daily Mail journalist, knew Gary well and set up a meeting. I remember a couple of days after we first went to discuss things, Gary sent me an email. It was headed: 'Ideas for a book – title undecided' and, in it, he proceeded to outline everything he had done in his career with a series of headings, and sub-headings, highlighting the main events.

That was Gary in a nutshell: someone who took pride in what he had done, and in everything he was doing; someone who made it easy for others, and someone who was generous with his time.

We would meet every week, for one to two hours at a time, and he'd talk me through the highs – and lows – of his career with searing honesty and, always, good humour. I'd deliver chapters when I'd finished them and he'd produce his red pen and go over them, scrawling down notes, corrections or suggestions. Or even things he'd subsequently recalled and wanted included. I think he found reminiscing about his life both therapeutic and also enjoyable.

Towards the end of our meetings, Gary would balance the tape recorder on his lap as he lay on the couch, his feet having swollen badly due to the medication and steroids he was on, but never once do I remember him complaining about things.

"Any gossip pal?" he'd invariably ask, anxious for any tit-bits I'd heard about Everton and Liverpool in my role as the Merseyside reporter for the Daily Express. He'd digest any information I could offer him, clearly missing being inside the game he loved so much.

When we met in early December to discuss his hopes for the future, and the plans he had drawn up to reach out to others, the book was effectively complete. However, we decided to leave the final pages until nearer the planned publication in April so that it would be as up to date as possible. Again, I began to understand that was Gary's way. Whatever he set out to do, he wanted it to be the best it could be.

I find it upsetting, now, when I re-read that final chapter, where Gary had outlined his intentions to speak at clubs and associations up and down the country and educate the next generation of sportsmen about his illness and what he had learned through 30 years in the game. He had plans, things he still wanted to do. He still hoped to return to management, something he had experienced only briefly with a cash-strapped Stockport County. When the end came, it felt abrupt and cruel, robbing him as it did of the aspirations to which he had still clung. But I still think it is important to detail the hopes Gary had, the things he still wanted to do. This wasn't a man who had given up, but someone I felt honoured to get to know.

Thanks go to Steve Hanrahan and Paul Dove from Sport Media for embracing the idea of the book so enthusiastically when Gary met them face-to-face, and for their advice in the months since. Thanks also to James Cleary on the production side.

To Dominic Fifield of The Guardian for his encouragement and, more importantly, persistence in tracking down a DVD of Gary's favourite game – a 5-2 Liverpool win at Stamford Bridge in December, 1989 – which Gary had spent years trying to get hold of and finally got to watch before Christmas.

And to Ged Rea for compiling the statistics and pointing out my mistakes.

There are lots of people who knew Gary better than I did, but I count myself as lucky to have spent time in his company and to have met his wife, Jacqueline, his children Scarlet, Reece and Riley and, more recently, Bella the bulldog.

This is Gary's story, a story he wanted to tell. I'm glad to have helped ensure that happened.

Paul Joyce, February 2012

Foreword by

Kenny Dalglish

People tell me I scored in the game in which Gary Ablett made his home debut for Liverpool, but I honestly can't remember that. Even now, though, I can picture Gary scoring that day. It was a well struck left-foot shot at the Anfield Road End past Steve Sutton as we beat Nottingham Forest 3-0. It was some way to make an impact. Some entrance. He set the standard early.

If it is possible to get local boys into the team then that is always preferable, but they cannot get in on their birthright. They have to get in because they deserve to on ability, and Gary made it by virtue of his talent at a time when the competition at Liverpool was fierce. That, alone, is testimony to his quality.

As a youngster, you always thought he had a chance. The problem he had was the people who were in front of him: Alan Hansen, Mark Lawrenson, Gary Gillespie, Jim Beglin, and then the likes of David Burrows and Steve Staunton. There was a lot of competition, but that brought out the best in Gary. In many ways, for a local boy, it is sometimes more difficult to be a success at a club like this, which makes the career he had all the more impressive.

Gary could do things better than some people in the team. Admittedly, other people had strengths he did not have, but we were in it together. We relied on him. He played in cup finals for us and helped us get to where we wanted to be as a club. As his manager, I knew his value and importance. I knew I could count on him.

The fact that he crossed over to the blue half of Merseyside and was accepted, after what was maybe a rough start, tells you something about the person as well. Not just his football ability, but the person. It is a strong character that moves between the two clubs, especially when they are born in the city. Other people have done it, but they weren't local lads. So the fact that he could regard himself as a success at both Liverpool and Everton speaks volumes: he had the ability to thrive as a player, and the qualities he needed to make his mark as a coach.

Gary came in to Melwood last October to visit us. The circumstances that brought him to us were sad, of course, but any of the former players are more than welcome to come in and watch the training. That is the way the football club should be. There should be an open door, within reason, for people to come in if they have been part of this football club. If they have been prepared to give their time to Liverpool, then it is the least we can do to give them a little bit of our time back, and show our appreciation.

The best thing about him coming in was that we all knew he wanted to be here. We didn't talk about the illness, not because we weren't interested but because he had done that enough. It was a day for him to bring his kids in, wander about the place and feel free to do what he wanted. He deserved our appreciation.

When I think of Gary, I think of someone who was brought up to be respectful by his parents, and someone who knew what was right and what was wrong, but that didn't take away any of the steely determination he had to make himself a footballer. He never shirked a challenge, on the pitch or off it.

Some people have a comfortable childhood and then think: "I'm okay. I don't need to do anything." But Gary was not one of them. To me, Gary Ablett worked hard and wanted that extra responsibility. He achieved success because of that.

It was a pleasure to have known him and to have worked with him. I think he can be very proud of what he did in his life.

Kenny Dalglish, February 2012

Foreword by

David Moyes

When I first came to Everton as manager, I didn't know an awful lot about Gary Ablett.

I knew him as a player obviously, and a successful one at that, but he was working as a youth coach at Everton when I arrived in March 2002, and there wasn't too much cross-over.

Over time what struck me about Gary was that apart from being well-mannered, he was always out watching and seeing what the first team was doing whenever he had a spare minute. That was how I got to know him a bit better really: through his eagerness to learn and improve himself.

I have to say that I was disappointed when he left Everton to join Liverpool in 2006, but it never really affected the relationship he had with people here. We weren't going to fall out because of that.

It says everything about the respect in which Gary was held that moving from Everton to Liverpool did not affect the relationships with the people who he left behind.

If Liverpool played Everton at reserve level, all the coaching staff would get on well and have a good time in each other's company. He actually called me when he was offered the Stockport job. He phoned me up and said he was excited about the opportunity. He wanted to take the job and give it a go.

I remember Gary asking about the young players we had at Everton and whether any of them could maybe link up with him in the future. That showed how his mind worked. He hadn't taken the job yet, but already he was thinking of ways of improving Stockport and giving them his total commitment.

He was definitely someone who was climbing the ladder of football management, trying to make the most of his talents as a coach. Everyone at Everton would only have good things to say, and good thoughts to have about him.

That was reflected when he fell ill.

Gary was coming into Finch Farm, and there was a period where he didn't look and feel great.

He didn't want to go into the cold, so he would sit in my office, which overlooks the training pitches, and he would watch the sessions. In many respects, he wasn't treated any differently to the coaches here. He'd sit and have a bit of lunch with the staff in the canteen, talking football and generally just mixing in.

When there was a great improvement in his condition, we were all excited and he actually came out and stood on the touchline a few times to watch training.

I was putting on the sessions and he'd be there at the side, studying everything. He was storing it away, ready to put into practice anything he thought was worthwhile for when he was back in the game.

It is a terrible shame that Gary should be denied that opportunity.

One of the things that comes to mind when I think about Gary is the way he would come into the training ground and he would say: "I'm fine, I'm good, I'm doing okay." He was incredible. We would sit and have a cup of tea together and I would be thinking to myself: 'How is he being so strong?' Most of us would curl up and not want to be seen. Gary was the opposite.

Sometimes you don't know what to say to people when they are ill, but Gary made it easy. He made everyone comfortable in his presence.

He was incredibly strong and didn't speak about himself, or what he was going through, but he was always interested in what was going on at Everton. He liked to talk football: what team we were going to play, how the youth team was doing, those sorts of things.

Right to the end, he was totally dignified. This was an illness where he knew there was a chance things might not work out, but the strength he showed, and the courage he had to keep fighting was fantastic.

It was terribly sad when he passed away. I had got the feeling in his last visits to Finch Farm that he was coming in and saying, 'Cheerio.' I desperately hoped that wasn't the case but, looking back, maybe that was Gary saying goodbye. He'd bring his boys, Riley and Reece, in and they are a credit to him and his family.

There are times in life where you weigh up what to do in certain situations. Sometimes you say to yourself, 'Och, I'll do that another day. Leave that until tomorrow.' When he was first diagnosed with cancer, I went to see Gary in hospital in Cambridge. I was nervous about going to see him, for whatever reason I don't really know.

Maybe it was because I can't say that I know him as well as some other people. But the decision to go and see him is one of those things that I am really pleased I did. It was uncomfortable at first, but I might never have had that moment with him otherwise.

If it helped Gary just a little bit then it was the least I could do.

David Moyes, February 2012

1
—

A Shock Result

It looked like I had been shot. There was blood everywhere. Bright red, fresh blood oozing from the puncture marks in my neck and hip, seeping out and staining the bed covers crimson.

A team of doctors and nurses had spent 20 minutes with their thumbs pressed down on the wounds, desperately trying to stem the bleeding. But here I was, almost as soon as they'd left, lying in a sea of red again.

The dressings to protect where I'd had two biopsies had not helped. They were soaked the same colour as my old Liverpool shirts. More pools of blood had formed on my hospital bed whenever I shuffled in the vain hope of trying to get more comfortable, the stains darkening as I squirmed.

I was a mess, barely able to comprehend what was happening to me. The last thing I needed was a nurse poking her head around the door to tell me, at around eight o'clock that Saturday night, that I had a visitor.

My first reaction was bemusement. Who would be visiting me? It couldn't be Jacqueline, my wife, because she had already been in to see me that day, spending hours at my bedside trying to keep my spirits up. Telling me everything would be okay, that things would improve.

I wondered if it might be another visit from Roy Keane, whose support had been phenomenal since I had fallen ill just weeks after taking up the offer to become part of his backroom staff at Ipswich Town.

Who else was there? Who else knew what was happening to me? After all, hardly anyone knew I'd been taken ill. From feeling so unwell that I had called the club doctor, to being admitted to hospital, to being blue lighted in an ambulance from Ipswich to Addenbrooke's in Cambridge: that had all passed in a blur. A whirlwind that had simply swept me along and dumped me here, in a bed, where I was a helpless figure in my own blood.

So you can imagine my surprise when the thin curtain that preserved some of my dignity from the rest of the patients on the ward was pulled aside and there was David Moyes poking his head through. My disbelief paled into insignificance compared to the shock he received.

He froze. His face dropped and straight away I could tell he didn't know what to say. Who would? He had just stumbled into a scene he could never have expected, something that would not have looked out of place on a battlefield.

Roy had called, informing him I had been taken ill. With Everton playing a pre-season friendly in nearby Norwich, David thought he would call in before he headed back to Merseyside.

He probably thought I would just be lying on a bed, looking a bit unwell, maybe off colour and drained. Perhaps, at worst, with a couple of drips attached to my arms.

He could never have envisaged pulling back the curtain to find someone who had worked as a youth coach under him at Everton lying in his own blood and in desperate, obvious need of help.

There was silence for a split second and then I muttered: "Er, could you give me five minutes to sort myself out."

"No problem, I'll go and get you a nurse," he replied, hastily drawing the curtain closed behind him and turning back out of the ward.

Had he carried on walking out of the hospital that would have been completely understandable. But, after the nurse tidied me up and applied new dressings, making me almost 'presentable', he came back in and we had a chat.

David's visit was a huge boost. He said everyone at Everton was thinking of me and praying for me, but it wasn't long before the conversation turned to football. What we know best. How pre-season was going, whether he'd be getting any more signings in, things like that. Everton had beaten Norwich City 4-2 that afternoon with a hat-trick from Tim Cahill, and David was really upbeat about his squad's chances for the season ahead.

It might seem strange to some people that, for the 20 minutes or so that he stayed, we chatted not so much about the illness – about the needle wounds that refused to stop oozing, or the course of treatment that would inevitably follow, or even about what might happen to me in the longer-term – but about the new season.

But at that stage I still believed I would be back at work in a couple of weeks. In any case, I could see David was awkward and uncomfortable at the state he'd found me in, and football was a common bond that we shared.

It was a bond that certainly did not involve hospitals, cancer and chemotherapy.

Up until July 22, 2010, I knew nothing of them, either. Of course, I know people whose relatives had suffered from this terrible disease, but my knowledge didn't go any deeper than that – it had no need to. I regarded myself as being fit and healthy, a football man, and I was looking forward to starting work for Roy.

I had been travelling back on the train home from Wokingham Park Hotel near Reading after doing a presentation for my FA Pro-Licence, alongside the likes of Aidy Boothroyd and Tony Mowbray, when Roy had called me.

He said there was a vacancy in his backroom team at Portman Road because one of his staff couldn't settle in the area, and he wanted to move back up to Nottingham. I already knew Antonio Gomez, the fitness coach at Ipswich Town, because he had worked at Liverpool with me and the reserves. When Roy asked if I'd be interested in the role, I jumped at the chance.

I'd not worked since leaving my first management job at Stockport County, and I didn't have any other options or offers.

"If you are asking me if I want the job, I will be there as soon as you need me," I told Roy.

That was on the Friday and by Sunday I was travelling down to East Anglia to start work. Ipswich put me up in a hotel, and I started work on the Monday. Everything was fine.

This was a challenge I needed, a route back into the game that had been my life and a job I relished, working with Roy and his team. He was someone who I had obviously admired as a player, and he had shown with Sunderland that he was cut out for management as well.

Ipswich were desperate to get back into the Premier League. Having Roy in charge, someone who lives for success, seemed the perfect fit. I couldn't wait to immerse myself and be part of things. Unfortunately, it was not going to be as straight forward as that.

I had been there for a week when I started to develop a couple of lumps, like boils, on my head. It was nothing for me to worry about, I thought. I'll get some pain killers, sleep things off and get back to my job as first-team coach.

I went to see Dr Steve Roberts, who was the club doctor, and he gave me some Ibuprofen to take. The lumps were itchy, angry and kind of sore. After the first one came out, there was a second and then a third. One of them ended up leaving a scar and making a little bit of a dent in my head that is still there today, covered by my hair.

The tablets took a bit of the sting out of things and I started to feel a little bit better. Panic over. It was probably all to do with the rush of coming down after taking the job and throwing myself straight into it. It was probably a reaction to a period of upheaval, and certainly nothing to be worried about.

Ipswich had played a couple of pre-season friendlies already before we went over to Eindhoven to play PSV one Saturday evening. But the night before, I just didn't feel right. I was tired, lethargic. I'd lost my appetite and was generally feeling under the weather.

It was as if I had all the symptoms of a flu, though the lumps on my head were a strange side-effect I could not explain.

I couldn't sleep that night, just lying awake hour after hour, worrying about what was wrong with me, but at the same time determined to make sure I was fine for the game, given that I'd just got the job. I wanted to impress.

We trained in the morning and played the game, which we lost 1-0, and then stayed over that night in Holland. I slept a little better, but by now I was becoming more concerned. There were new symptoms emerging. My head was still sore, but now my teeth and gums hurt. I was still lethargic, feeling drained and run down. It would not have been so bad, but I'd never really had any of the symptoms all at once before. I couldn't put my finger on why they were happening to someone who had been fit and healthy enough to have played football almost every day of his life since he had been 16.

I flew home with the team and when we arrived back on the Sunday lunchtime, Roy gave us two days off. I drove back to Tarleton, not far from Southport, where Jacqueline and my three kids, Scarlet, Reece and Riley, were still living.

I told Jacqueline that I wasn't feeling well, but she knew. Usually I am someone who is always on the go all the time and it is unlike me to want to sleep in the day, but just lifting my head off the pillow for two days was a struggle. I just wanted to be in bed, sleep off what I presumed was a virus and then I'd be okay.

But at the end of the couple days I'd had off, I felt no better and Jacqueline badgered me to go and get myself checked out by a doctor.

"I'll see Dr Roberts when I get to Ipswich," I assured her, before driving down to the Milsoms Hotel where I was staying in Suffolk. The journey, all five hours of it, drained me completely. I got into the hotel, went to bed and that was me.

There was no way I could get into work. Not a chance. So I rang to tell them and made my excuses, worrying that this wasn't the impression that Roy would have wanted his new boy to make.

My concerns were daft really because if anyone had seen me, they would have known straight away that I wasn't in any fit state to be putting players through their paces when I could barely summon the energy to walk myself.

I was all over the place, and didn't know why. I started retching and vomiting. I couldn't eat properly – nothing would stay down, and my appetite had vanished anyway. My eyes had hemorrhaged and were bloodshot, and it was a battle to pick up the telephone in my room and return calls to speak to Jacqueline.

It wasn't long before she'd had enough.

She took the kids out of school and they all came down, although I wish they'd not been confronted by the sight that greeted them.

I was like a zombie, groping my way to the hotel room door to let my family in, then shuffling pathetically back to bed. I had no energy left, I had nothing.

As soon as she saw me, she called the club and was told I should come down for some blood tests. Somehow, with Jacqueline's help, I made it from the hotel to the car, then from the car to the doctor's surgery before just flopping in a chair, seven sheets to the wind.

I don't think the kids realised what was happening but, then again, I was none the wiser. They waited outside while I went in for the blood tests with Jacqueline, and I can remember the doctor shaking and studying the vial of blood for what seemed like ages.

"Is everything ok?" Jacqueline asked.

The doctor said that something wasn't right, and I think it was then that Jacqueline started to have an inkling that this wasn't a virus and that it could be more serious than that. Me? I was still oblivious to everything, though that was soon to change.

Dr Roberts said he wanted to book us into hospital and do some more tests, and we got a call the following day to come down to Ipswich Hospital because a bed had become available.

We were told to report to one ward in particular and so, after we'd parked up, we started following the signs. Dragging myself up the steps at the old Wembley Stadium to collect a loser's medal after Liverpool had lost to Wimbledon back in 1988 hadn't been pleasant, but that was a stroll in the park compared to what followed that afternoon.

We walked down what seemed like a never-ending corridor, seeing signs for all the different wards and units you'd expect to find in a hospital, all the ones that you might spend a night on or, at worst, a couple of days. Neurology, occupational therapy, there was a sign for the hospital's chapel.

There was nothing much more. But we were walking on and becoming increasingly aware that, the deeper we went into the hospital, the more seriously ill the patients appeared to be getting.

"Where are we going here?" I asked Jacqueline but, with every step, I was starting to come to my senses a little bit more, jolted out of my trance-like state by the growing fear and realization of where this was headed. The increasingly frightened look on my wife's face served to shrug me awake as well.

Eventually we arrived at Oncology and the nurse took me into a little ward. There were about six beds in it and all the patients, all male, were wired up to various machines. They were older than me, some of them considerably older. A few of them looked frail, gaunt and they had turned a yellow-ish colour.

We sat on the bed and I turned to Jacqueline and said: "Don't worry. They've found us a bed. I'm here for some tests.

"That's all, and then we'll be away. One night at most while they do what they have to do."

But, even then, I'm pretty sure we were both wondering whether we were kidding ourselves.

The nurse or the sister who was on duty came over and asked if everything was alright. Maybe she sensed that we looked perplexed, as we were petrified.

"No, not really," I said. "I've been told to come here, but that's all. I haven't been told anything other than that I'm having some further tests. What's going on?"

"So you don't know why you are here?" she said.

"No."

She looked surprised, and it was then that my world collapsed.

"I'm sorry to have to tell you this, but we have found a really aggressive form of non-Hodgkin's lymphoma and if we don't treat it right now, you could be in trouble," she said.

And that was that. A life-changing sentence uttered matter of factly, like a manager reading out his starting XI at half past one on a Saturday afternoon.

Cancer.

I had cancer.

It's only now that I understand why she didn't dress it up with rather more sympathy. It's just part of her job; she has to remain detached from things, stay apart from those she's helping to treat. But, for us, it was upsetting as though our world had caved in. Devastating. The abruptness, the shock... well, it felt as if I had been punched.

Floored.

Cancer.

I went to pieces.

Why me?

How can this be happening to me?

Ever since I fell ill the slightest thing has set me off, but back then it just wasn't like me to cry.

It's not a very 'football' way to react to things, after all. But that day I wept buckets, with Jacqueline in floods of tears at my side.

2

—

Fighting Back

I knew I didn't have a virus now, but an illness that could kill me. Even so, I didn't really know what lymphoma was. Only that it wasn't good. The full gravity of the illness would become clear to me soon enough: lymphoma is a cancer of the lymphatic cells of the immune system.

There was no hanging around. I had a bone marrow biopsy which they took from just around by my hip, but I was only in Ipswich for one night because they said they didn't have the staff, or the consultants, who were specialised enough in the seriousness of the illness I had contracted. Instead, I was referred to Addenbrooke's over in Cambridge.

There I came under the guidance of Dr George Fellows, a specialist in his field and someone who explained better what was happening to me. By now, the right side of my face and the lymph glands in my neck had swollen up like footballs. I looked a proper state, but was numb to what was going on – helpless in my state of shock. The doctors there took another biopsy, this time from my neck, and I just accepted what was happening. I could hardly get my head around any of it, anyway. Even getting the biopsies served as a crash course in medical procedures for me that I wish I'd never have had. First of all they froze the area, the hip or the neck, and then pressed what was rather like a gun into the flesh.

A needle darted in and then back out to get a sample. This happened four or five times. It was sore and it was from these puncture marks that I would later start bleeding from my neck.

I'd sit there, desperate for it all to end, but desperate too for them to find out exactly what was going on. Maybe the biopsies would provide proper answers? But these procedures made it all seem more real.

The ward I was put on in Addenbrooke's was very similar to the one at Ipswich, but with one huge difference. The patients here looked as though they were suffering more than those I had spent a night with before. Their illnesses were more serious. There was a young lad to my right in the first bed, but again everyone else was older than me. You nod, you say hello. But there it ends. I'm quite a private person and I wouldn't open up easily. I just thought: 'They have their own problems, so why do they want to speak to me?'

It was around this time, while I was still taking in my new surroundings, that we decided to tell the children, or rather Jacqueline told them. She had befriended a lymphoma nurse at Ipswich – not the one who had first told us I had cancer, I should add – and she said it was right to tell the kids what was happening.

But how do you tell three children who were under the age of 15 that their dad has cancer? I don't know. It was left to Jacqueline because such was the speed with which I had been whisked away to Addenbrooke's in an ambulance that they were all left behind at the hospital in Ipswich. Like everything else since my life changed, she did it with such strength and devotion.

The kids were taken into a side room with Jacqueline and Jon

Walters, who was at Ipswich at the time but who now plays for Stoke. Jon's from the Wirral and when I first came down to East Anglia to link up with Roy's squad, we'd hit it off immediately, probably because of the Liverpool connection. He was fantastic, ferrying Jacqueline around Ipswich because she didn't know the area at all, taking her and the kids to the hospital.

Jon had lost his mother at a young age to bowel cancer, and said he had wished he'd been told about the gravity of the situation at the time. He could relate to what the kids were going to be going through, so he sat in with them.

He didn't need to do that, but it summed up the way most people at Ipswich were when I fell ill. They couldn't do too much. They were brilliant. I'm forever thankful to Jon for what he did that day.

Jacqueline later told me that the children had a right good whinge for about 10 minutes or so when she explained what was happening to me, but after that they were okay. They deal with things in their own way, but when people say I've been brave I always think to what they've been through, too.

It's asking a lot of children to get their heads around something as serious as this, but the way they have dealt with everything has been inspirational to me.

I suppose it was fortunate in a way that we did decide to tell them straight away because when Jacqueline left the hospital her attention was drawn to billboards outside a newsagents.

'Town coach in cancer shock,' they screamed. Soon it was all over Facebook as well. Nothing is private any more.

The Saturday that David Moyes came to visit, a couple of days after I had first been admitted to Addenbrooke's, was the first day I had started bleeding. The following day was the worst. My blood would not clot properly.

It was Scarlet's 15th birthday and just to make matters worse, all the family were coming down the corridor and onto the ward to see me when they overheard one of the nurses on the telephone, asking the doctors for more help because they simply couldn't stop the bleeding.

Panic set in. They were ushered into a room for half-an-hour while the medics tried to sort me out, patching me up so that I could see them and celebrate with my daughter, but you can imagine the upset they went through. It wasn't the birthday Scarlet wanted or deserved.

To be honest, I tried to keep the visits from the kids to a minimum. Jacqueline would spend three or four hours at a time at the hospital, but I didn't want the children on the ward for that long. Hospitals aren't places for kids, let alone a cancer ward with their dad stretched out in front of them, having to undergo four transfusions due to the amount of blood lost and three or four bags of platelets to try and get the blood to coagulate. There are some things a child shouldn't see, even if I was so desperate always to spend as much time with them as I possibly could.

Thankfully, Addenbrooke's is so big that there's even a shopping complex attached. The kids would go and look in the shops, sometimes with their grandmother, just so that they weren't sat around waiting. That kept them preoccupied, distracted. Even if it did my credit card no good in the long run!

After a few days the doctors managed to stop the bleeding and, because of the sheer volume of people who had started to come and visit, they moved me to another room.

My mum and dad, Roslyn and Neil, had come down from Liverpool and were staying in a bed and breakfast in Cambridge. John Ward, who was the Colchester United manager at the time but was someone I had worked with at Stockport, popped in to visit.

There was also Hughie McAuley, the former Liverpool youth coach. I knew Hughie well – he had also worked under me at Stockport County. He had been on holiday in Cheltenham with his wife Maria when he found out I was ill. Straight away he jumped in his car and drove the two hours or so to Cambridge to see me.

Hughie stayed for about four hours and we talked about anything and everything. Some people don't like to linger too much on what you are going through simply because they don't feel comfortable having that sort of conversation, but Hughie was interested in the medical side of it all and what treatments I was having. By the end, he left with enough information that lymphoma could be his specialised subject if he ever went on 'Mastermind'.

We talked about Liverpool, too, and what was happening there. Rafa Benitez had lost his job with Roy Hodgson taking over, while the Tom Hicks and George Gillett ownership of the club was going into meltdown. But we also talked about the old days: about some of the characters who used to be at the club like Jimmy Aspinall, the legendary scout who spotted me as a kid; about scoring on my Anfield debut.

Those moments are precious. The unexpected visits meant so much and for a time, maybe if only for a few seconds, you do forget where you are and why you are there in hospital. Then – inevitably, cruelly – it all comes rushing back.

I remember the first day of the 2010/11 season. That was the day I should have been making my presence felt among Roy Keane's backroom staff, taking my first steps back into the professional game after my experiences at Stockport.

But, instead, I was lying in a hospital bed, with my only chance of immersing myself in the game I love effectively reduced to me waiting for 'Match of the Day' or any football to come on the mini-TV I had in my room.

It was strange for me not to be involved in a new campaign, not to be basking in that familiar sense of optimism you have each year in August, that the season is going to end up in glory, a promotion party or something even better.

It is such a mouth-watering afternoon, normally, and something that you've waited all summer to come around. But, rather than being in the dug-out at the Riverside up on Teesside, I'd been left back on a Cambridge hospital ward waiting for all the Championship results to come in on 'Final Score'. Even though I felt out of it, I was thrilled when I heard Ipswich had won 3-1 at Middlesbrough.

Boro had spent a lot of money on the likes of Kris Boyd, Scott McDonald, Kevin Thomson and Stephen McManus, and were favourites to win the title and return to the Premier League, so it was a great result for the boys.

I was chuffed to bits for them and Roy. The season had started as the club meant to go on.

But my own evening rather dragged as I waited to catch a glimpse of some goals, and it must have been about 9.30pm when there was a knock on my door and a face appeared, squeezed up against the window. It was Roy.

"Are you ok, Gary?" he mouthed through the glass.

"Yes, yes, come in, come in," I said. "How did the team play?"

As he was opening the door, he said: "I've brought a few of the staff, I hope that's ok?"

I was made up. Antonio Gomez walked in, with Ian 'Charlie' McParland, Tony Loughlan, Matt Byard the physio and James 'Jimbo' Hollman, the goalkeeping coach.

Now the room admittedly had an en suite, but it still wasn't very big. It already felt a bit squeezed with the coaching staff all there, but next Jon Walters walked in and shook my hand, to be followed by Mark Kennedy, Grant Leadbitter, Carlos Edwards... until 18 or 19 lads, plus all the coaches were in the room with me. They were all crammed in there like sardines.

The team had flown back to Cambridge after the win, and Roy had said to them all that he wanted them to pop in and see me.

Now after the result they had just enjoyed I am sure a few of the lads fancied a night out – not that they were ever going to say 'no' to Roy – so this wasn't what they had in mind. I could also see that some of them felt uncomfortable.

After all, I had only been at the club a few weeks and a lot of the lads didn't really know me. Add to that the fact that my neck had ballooned up as well, and I didn't look the best, well it was only natural that a few of them must have wondered what they were doing here.

They stayed for about 10 minutes, during which time I tried to have a laugh with some of them, but to be honest it was just so hard for me to stop myself from bursting into tears.

It was all very emotional, but it speaks volumes for the way Ipswich Town Football Club does things, and the story serves as a measure of the man that Roy is. Later the players at Ipswich had a collection for me. They raised £9,000 to put towards a holiday for the family or something like that. Such generosity went beyond the call. I was overwhelmed. They didn't need to do that.

Roy has this reputation as a hard man, hard as nails, and detached emotionally. But I have seen another side to him with the support he's constantly offered me throughout my illness. Most weeks I get a call from him, or a text, asking how I'm doing. Sometimes if he is in Manchester he will come across to the house and visit. Another time he drove up from Ipswich with the staff in tow.

That visit was a huge boost for me at the time, and it must have contributed to the progress I started to make in my rehabilitation. I had started a course of chemotheraphy called R-CHOP.

R-CHOP is named after the initials of the drugs that you receive, four separate ones with complex sounding names like Rituximab, Cyclophosphamide, Doxorubicin and Vincristine. You also have Prednisolone tablets to take.

The nurse inserts a thin tube called a cannula into a vein in your hand, which is uncomfortable in itself. Once the chemotheraphy is ready, you are given anti-sickness drugs to combat the side-effects.

The first dose of Rituximab enters slowly into the bloodstream as an infusion over four hours, and then the other drugs follow.

It's a tiring, slow process, and I had one session as an inpatient and one as an out-patient because the doctors had become impressed by my progress.

I had been in Addenbrooke's for three weeks, when they said I could go back to the hotel the family were in, and even added that there was a chance I might be able to go back to work one or two days a week.

As distressing as being told you have lymphoma is, this was massive. I had something to aim for now, a return to work. Hearing the doctors say that was huge.

'I'm going to be alright,' I thought. It was as if all the upset, trauma and heartache of the past few weeks would seem like a bad dream.

But, with cancer, you can never get ahead of yourself.

I'd gone back to the hotel, my life taking on aspects of normality again – well, to a small degree I suppose, and I even went to watch Ipswich's reserves play Stevenage one afternoon. I took Riley along for some company. It was windy and horrible, the sort of day you look out of the window at and want to clear up.

But I was out and about watching football, feeling a bit more like I was part of the game again. It had served to whet my appetite and had me dreaming of going back to work full-time, getting back on the coaching pitches and into the dug-out, and proving to Roy and the team that I'd been a worthy appointment.

When I got home that night, Jacqueline asked if my face was okay.

"Yes. Why?"

She said it just didn't look right and, sure enough, as the night wore on, my face gradually started to droop. I had developed a condition called Bell's Palsy, which is a type of facial paralysis that ends up leaving your face sagging.

I'd been warned about some of the side-effects of chemotherapy; flu-like symptoms for one and flushing, but not this.

A day on which I'd started harbouring hopes of returning to work, ended up with me undergoing an MRI scan and, potentially, having suffered a significant set-back in my recovery. The implications, again, took a while to sink in.

Dr Fellows called me back into his surgery, once the MRI scan results had come in and, throughout the conversation on Bell's Palsy, there was a lymphoma nurse present as well, which hadn't happened at any of the chats we'd had before. I started to get nervous, but kept telling myself I'd be back at work soon, coaching again.

Then Dr Fellows dropped the bombshell, inadvertently of course, that he was actually glad I'd suffered the Bell's Palsy. Without it, he said, they might not have performed the tests which showed the cancer had penetrated into my spinal fluid. There was a chance that the illness would spread to my brain.

His words were like a sledgehammer. From geeing myself up about being back on the training pitch the week before, now here I was being told the cancer might spread to my brain. If it had, what chance would there be of making a recovery? I sat in the chair shell-shocked. Never mind going back to work: was I actually going to survive this illness?

It was decided to increase the aggressiveness of the chemotherapy treatment. Dr Fellows explained that it wasn't worth me undergoing the treatment down in Cambridge, given how far it was from Tarleton, and suggested, if only for my peace of mind, that I moved back up north.

I'd be treated instead at The Christie Hospital in Manchester, which had been recommended to me by the referee Mark Halsey. I didn't know Mark particularly well, but he got in touch with me after his own successful fight against throat cancer and just said to me that this was the best hospital in Europe for the treatment I was going to need. He suggested I called an oncologist called Professor Tim Illidge – an Everton fan, as it happened, and someone who was happy to see me and talk over the treatment.

I was expecting to be treated privately. I had been offered a contract by Ipswich, which I agreed to sign. The CEO, Simon Clegg, was going away on holiday for a fortnight and the i's would be dotted and t's crossed when he returned.

It was in that two-week window, however, that I fell ill.

On the morning I was due to start my treatment, I got in touch with Ipswich and they said I wasn't covered because I hadn't actually put pen-to-paper yet.

In my opinion that was wrong. I felt that as soon as I had agreed the deal, the medical cover should have started. It wasn't my fault the CEO had gone away. I have to say that Simon has since been very good to me, sorting out some insurance paperwork, but at the time I felt badly let down.

The impression I had was that going private would be better for me, with a superior level of care and higher quality of food. But I spoke to Tim and he said as far as he was concerned, there would be no difference in the standard of treatment I'd receive. For a few hundred pounds more, I might have a room with some oak pannelling in it, but as for the care, it would be the same.

In fact, he felt I would get better care in the Haematology Transplant Unit at The Christie because it is more of an isolation unit. I have been treated there ever since and the staff have been outstanding.

I've certainly kept them busy.

One of the consequences of contracting Bell's Palsy, and my face falling, was that my eye wouldn't close. We literally had to tape the eyelid down, and more so in the evening, because the doctors didn't want my eye to dry out – then I would have been in even more trouble.

I had gel to put in it to try and keep the eye moist, and by the time I next saw Tim I was a bag of shite again.

We gave him a brief outline of my case and he said it wasn't his area of expertise, but recommended me to see Dr Adrian Bloor instead.

He was straight with me. He said I had to be prepared for what might be a very bumpy road ahead, and that he didn't have a crystal ball to see into the future.

But that was enough.

For the first month I had been quite negative about everything and quite down. You start thinking: why me? How, when I played for Liverpool and Everton, two of the biggest clubs in the world as far as I was concerned, can this be happening to me? Then you sort of go into denial and look for someone to blame, which is daft.

Eventually, I accepted that it had nothing to do with apportioning blame and that it could happen to anyone, whether you are the fittest person in the world or not. If it's your time, it's your time. Cancer does not discriminate.

So you have to make a decision. What are you going to do? Are you going to feel sorry for yourself, constantly bemoaning how unfair life has been dealing you these cards. Or, do you make some positive choices as to how you are going to take your life forward?

I knew the answer because there is no other choice.

3

First Impressions

There is nothing that can prepare you for the fight against cancer. When the diagnosis is delivered you're left numb. When you eventually come around, you're scared witless. It takes time to mentally accept what is happening to you, and dare to face the future. But perhaps in a small way, the fact that I had faced so many challenges in my career helped me realise that this was simply another fight, albeit one that was far more serious than I had previously experienced. A fight that I had to win.

Few footballers have a seamless rise to prominence, and setting out on a career that took me from Liverpool, via Derby County and Hull City, to Everton, then on to Sheffield United, Birmingham City, Wycombe Wanderers with my old friend Lawrie Sanchez, and then Blackpool, it became clear that whenever I cleared one hurdle, another would spring up right in front of me.

All along the way, I had to push to get noticed. As a starry-eyed youngster I faced a struggle even to be taken seriously: a battle to prove to the teachers, who shook their heads and said I was making a huge mistake when I left school to pursue a career in football, that they were wrong. And, just as significantly, a constant battle to show Liverpool that they shouldn't turn my dreams to dust before I had even had a chance to realise them.

Back when I was starting out, it was Tuesday and Thursday nights, not Saturday afternoons, around which my world revolved. I'd finish school and get the 61 bus from Aigburth Vale to West Derby – the fare was about 50p – twice a week to Liverpool's training ground, Melwood, and train under the watchful eye of youth coach John Bennison.

When you walked out on those pitches you felt 10ft tall even though, at that stage, I was still small and quite chubby. It was the start of a dream I hoped would catapult me into the first team, playing in front of 45,000 fans and a throbbing Kop for, what I considered to be, the best team on the planet.

Training was against other young hopefuls who were either the same age or older than me. The likes of Paul Jewell, Mark Seagraves, Tony Kelly, Howard Gayle and Jimmy Comer – who is the masseur at Everton these days – used to go down to Melwood, each of them trying to catch the eye of the coaches. Pulling on a red jersey and playing at Anfield was the ultimate goal, but all of us had a more immediate aim in mind back then.

Melwood was basic with none of the state-of-the-art facilities the Liverpool players enjoy now. There was no canteen or swimming pool, and no media room. It was more or less a small pavilion with a couple of changing rooms and a few side rooms.

The objective on a Tuesday was to do well enough in training so that, when you returned two days later on the Thursday, the coaches would remember you and select you to play on the staff team. Thursday was when first-team coaches Ronnie Moran and Roy Evans came down, forgetting the senior side and the likes of Kenny Dalglish and Graeme Souness for a bit, and joining in with the kids who one day hoped to emulate their heroes.

There wasn't a trophy to play for, but believe me those Thursday night games were the be all and end all back then. You were desperate to show Ronnie and Roy you could play the Liverpool way – pass and move, pass and move – and that you were one to keep an eye on, the player that caught the eye. You were basically on trial every week. A bad session and you went home in bits. Do okay and you felt you'd made a name for yourself.

All day at St Margaret's School, Aigburth, I would think of nothing else but trying to impress the coaches, especially Ronnie. He was the driving force that made Liverpool so competitive, the man who would leave the first team's championship medals in a cardboard box for the likes of Kenny, Alan Hansen and Graeme to root out themselves, rather than stand to receive on ceremony. He was not one for creating a scene. The past was the past for Ronnie, all he was bothered about was doing things better the next time.

I hated not being on the staff side on a Thursday and, more often than not, I used to get picked for them. If it seems unfair that the staff picked the players who had stuck in their memory, then that's because I think it was designed so that the staff always won. There were times when the staff team had fewer players in a bid to even things up, but they'd still run out winners.

Roy had a great touch and would run around a bit, but Ronnie would get it and lay it off, keeping it simple. Pass and move, pass and move. Practising what he preached to the first team. You'd get the ball and play it into Ronnie, and then look to support him. You were desperate to make your passes perfect, striving to make a constant impression, and you certainly didn't want him bawling at you in front of the other lads.

One Thursday I'd been picked for the staff team again and was just concentrating on doing what I did every other week. Keep the ball moving, try not to give the ball away, move into space, find your man, support the player on the ball.

"Here! I'm fucking here, not over there," barked Ronnie, sending a shudder right through me. Concentrate, I thought to myself. Come on. It's just one mistake. Just don't make another. Head down, concentrate.

However, what I thought was one mistake soon, in Ronnie's eyes at least, became two, three, four, five, six. The messages were straight to the point: "Shite." "Don't run there, find some bloody space." "You've stopped. What have you fucking stopped for?"

I got an absolute pasting off him. Nothing I did was right. When I played the ball into him, instead of "well done, son" like normal, there was a bollocking. When I made a run, it was always into the wrong area of the pitch.

"What was that? What the fuck are you doing?"

Time after time after time again. It was 45 minutes of absolute torture. I have to say it wasn't personal abuse, all of it was football related, but that didn't make things any easier to bear. I wanted the earth to swallow me up.

I kept my gob shut. You never said anything back to Ronnie. Can you imagine a snotty-nosed schoolboy picking a fight with the first-team coach of Liverpool, someone who had played for the club, worked under Bill Shankly, Bob Paisley and now Joe Fagan? Someone who, at that time, had been on the touchline in Rome '77, Wembley '78, Paris '81? The scenes of the club's greatest achievements. There was no answering back.

The session ended and I walked off dejected, thinking: 'That's it. That's me finished at Liverpool.' I didn't want to make eye contact with any of the other lads who had witnessed my humiliation. Head down, stare at the ground, get out of there. I'd not been handed an apprenticeship yet and this was clearly their way of breaking the news to me that I wouldn't be receiving one. They'd obviously watched me and I wasn't measuring up to what they wanted. I was distraught. This felt like the end.

You used to get your expenses on a Thursday from Tom Saunders, another wise old member of the Anfield think-tank that kept Liverpool out in front. It was £2.50, which would cover the bus fares and leave enough for a bag of chips on the way home. As I traipsed off I just wanted to get home. Get to the chippie and drown my sorrows.

Then I felt this arm on my shoulder. It was Roy.

"What do you think?" he asked.

"I don't know what to think," I mumbled, shaking my head. "I've tried to do the same things that I have been doing for the past 12 months. I just don't understand what I've done wrong."

There was a silence for a few seconds, and then Roy came clean.

"Ronnie was testing you," he said. "We were looking for someone to keep going, someone with a bit of the 'I'll show you' attitude. What we didn't want was someone who goes into their shell and can't perform when the pressure is on, when not everything is going right. That's not the type of player we want at Liverpool."

From feeling like my hopes had crashed and burned, things were looking up again. I started to understand what the previous tongue-lashing had been about. Unwittingly, perhaps, I'd passed the test.

Ronnie, of course, said nothing to me. He was the bad cop and Roy the good cop. It had been difficult not to let my head drop as the abuse had rained down on me, but in those situations you have to drive yourself on. I'm sure the other lads had gone through something similar, but you don't notice so much when it is not directed at you.

It was every man for himself because everyone wanted the same thing – everyone knew what was at stake. What we didn't know was how many apprenticeships would be given out, if any at all. My age group was a particularly poor year, so the worry was that Liverpool might not take anyone on. It nagged away at you all the time.

What Ronnie did wouldn't be allowed today given how the country has become so politically correct, especially because his abuse had been directed at someone who was still a minor. But, while I hated it at the time, it didn't do me any harm in the long-run. The kids today are over-protected, in my opinion. Having worked since as a youth coach at Everton and as reserve-team manager at Liverpool, I'm better placed than most to say that the teenagers that come through the ranks are mollycoddled.

They don't learn the trade as we once did and, half the time, they don't even come into contact with the first-team players anymore. The first team at Liverpool and the academy operate off different sites, at Melwood and in Kirkby, and while everyone is on one complex with Everton at Finch Farm, there still isn't enough crossover. While I grew up at the school of hard knocks, the youngsters today have nothing to worry about except playing football. All clubs have Child Welfare and Education Officers now to make sure the young players are catered for, whatever the problems. Times have changed since I was given that public ear-bashing, but things like that served to toughen me up.

It seems strange to think of it now, but even before Ronnie and Liverpool got hold of me and set about trying to whip me into shape, I could have been pulling on a red shirt for a different team. I was 14 coming up to 15, when I was asked by Manchester United to go for a week's trial there.

Joe Armstrong, who was the United scout for the Liverpool area, approached my dad and said that I'd spend a week in halls of residence at Salford University, and go to the old Cliff training complex each day to play a game.

I'd started going to Liverpool games with my dad and, while I knew the rivalry with United was huge, I thought it was still worthwhile going. I hadn't signed for anyone at this point and, as much as I longed for Liverpool to show an interest in me, there was no guarantee, at that stage, that they ever would. If things didn't work out for me with Liverpool, maybe they would somewhere else.

The one thing I knew was that I wanted to be a professional footballer, so I had no real qualms about going to other teams on trial. Even to the enemy – United.

It's an outlook that stood me in good stead later in my career. You have to be pragmatic as a player and be prepared to go where you are wanted. Football is many things, but it is never predictable and only a few players see their careers pan out exactly as they envisaged they would. Or, indeed, how they wanted them to.

I'd been to trials far and wide. I went to Derby County for a day, Blackburn for a day. I played in a trial match for them in midfield and came home. I didn't do anything out of the ordinary, but at the same time I didn't do anything wrong. Just okay. At United, I'd have more time to impress, a week of trials where I could show them properly what I could do. Or so I thought.

After half-an-hour, I wanted to come home. Of all the lads who had been invited along, United had made the mistake of not making sure they had picked two goalkeepers. The 20 outfield players were selected and when I wasn't one of them, I knew what was coming.

"Would you mind going in goal?" asked one of the coaches.

I agreed because I thought it was the right thing to do – you don't kick up a fuss when you're on trial at a club like United – but, from that moment, my mind was made up. I wouldn't be signing for United even if, during the rest of the week, I stood out like a beacon.

Maybe that is one of the reasons why United lagged behind Liverpool at that stage, embroiled in a constant game of catch up that Liverpool fans can now appreciate, with roles having been reversed.

If their approach to recruitment was such that they didn't even invite two goalkeepers to a week of trials, it was little wonder they were in the doldrums. It was amateurish. I was expecting everything there to be slick and professional.

It took the shine off the trial. I let a few in, of course, but what did they expect? Back then, I saw myself as a central midfielder, occasionally a striker for my Sunday League side, St Michael's, and certainly not a goalkeeper. I wanted to be dictating the tempo of the trial and doing well enough, so that if United were to offer me schoolboy terms word might get back to Liverpool as well, and jolt them into life. To be denied that chance was depressing. Utterly depressing. I stuck out the week, and eventually got the chance to show what I could do in midfield, because I thought it was the right thing to do. How would it look if I stormed off after one day?

But the whole experience was an eye-opener for what was to come later in my career. A reality check, a reminder that life in football wasn't going to be about turning up and expecting to be given the chance to play in my favourite position. There were going to be obstacles flung down in front of me at every turn.

At the end of the week, United said they would be in touch. They never were, but there wouldn't have been any point. I'd never play for them. With each passing day, I was being swayed towards Liverpool.

Everton had never been in touch, but Liverpool's interest had been mentioned to my dad through the scout Jimmy Aspinall and then John Bennison. Even now, I can remember John coming round to my parents' house in Latrigg Road, Aigburth Vale, with what I suppose you could call a 'bung'.

It wasn't a bundle of cash, an envelope stuffed full of notes, or the promise of a house and a job for a relative as is often the case now. Instead, he presented me with a pair of shorts and one of the heavy duty, black woolly jumpers that the first team used to wear in training.

"We'd like you to come in and train with us twice a week," said John. "We think you've got something and that you'd be better coming to Liverpool than anywhere else."

Before he had even finished speaking I was thinking: 'Deal.'

In my head, the shorts belonged to Kenny Dalglish and the knitted jumper was one of Graeme Souness' but, to be honest, the gifts weren't necessary. Liverpool wanted me. That was enough. When do I begin?

It was the start of a dream. The dream I'd had when I used to jump on the back of my dad's moped, stick on a crash helmet and go with him to the police club on Prescot Road, Fairfield, every Saturday.

Sport ran in the family. My great grandfather, Tommy, played for Tranmere Rovers and while Jessie Owens was winning gold at the 1936 Olympics in Berlin, my grandfather Les was helping Great Britain to a commemorative medal in the Water Polo.

My other grandad, Jimmy, also had the claim to fame of having played in the same Durham Light Infantry team as the legendary Bill Nicholson, who led Tottenham to the Double in 1961.

And my dad could have played professionally, too. He had a good left foot and could have had a career himself as a midfielder with Burnley, but chose instead to go into the police because of the job security.

I was about seven when I used to go and watch him play with the police team. They'd put the nets up and go in to get changed, leaving me to stay on the pitch smashing a ball into the goal before the match. I'd reluctantly come off at kick-off, but only to see if I could find anyone else who wanted a kick about. That's all that I wanted to do.

My love for Liverpool grew when I started going to Anfield. I remember the first time we went ended in disappointment. It was the European Cup quarter-final against St Etienne in 1977, and the ground was packed. We walked around and around the stadium trying to get a ticket, but to no avail. My dad even showed his Police ID on one of the gates in an attempt to persuade one of the stewards to let us in, but they were probably tired of the sob stories they'd been hearing for hours by then. So, we were stranded outside the night David Fairclough scored his memorable goal against the French side to propel Liverpool into the semi-finals, en route to their first European Cup success.

To make up for missing out on one of the club's most glorious nights, we went to see Liverpool play Middlesbrough in an FA Cup quarter-final a few days later. Liverpool won 2-0 thanks to goals from Fair-clough, again, and Kevin Keegan, in front of a huge crowd of 55,881. It was magical being inside Anfield for the first time. Keegan was one of my idols growing up, a mantle Kenny Dalglish took on when he was signed to replace him later that year, and I was drawn to everything he did. Yes, he could score goals, but he also worked so hard. He was someone intent on squeezing every last drop out of his talent. A role model, I thought.

But my abiding memory of that occasion was not of the goals, but of Jimmy Case having Graeme Souness, who was still at Boro then, by the throat in the middle of the pitch. They had been niggling at each other throughout the game before tensions finally boiled over. I think Jimmy knew he had met his match pretty quickly, and I am sure he was made up when we signed Graeme the following season.

I turned to my dad and he was just smiling as if to say: "Those are two real men, son. Everyone wants to win, but who wants it more?"

It wasn't just on the pitch that we'd witness wanton violence. I remember Chelsea coming to Anfield. They used to put all the away fans in the right-hand corner of the Anfield Road End as you look at it from the Kop. We were in the middle section behind the goal getting ready for the game, when the Chelsea supporters came storming up the stairs straight into the Liverpool section and everyone scattered. They put the fear of God into everyone. They'd come looking to cause trouble, but everyone just vanished. For a young kid, that was an eye-opener. The other side of football. The ugly side.

But the fact that, not long after I'd started attending Anfield as a supporter, I was playing there for Liverpool's youth team merely fuelled my dreams further.

I was still at school at the time, and playing centre-forward on a Sunday for St Michael's in Jericho Lane. One weekend I scored nine, and John Bennison asked if I'd like to come and be on the bench for an FA Youth Cup tie with Manchester United at Old Trafford. There was no need to ask twice. This was massive, a real step up on my learning curve and, of course, the chance of gaining a level of revenge on United. Maybe I would get a chance to show them that I might not have been a good goalkeeper, but as an outfield player I wasn't too bad.

It was the first time I had come across Mark Hughes and Norman Whiteside, and others like Graeme Hogg. They lined up against us that day and what struck me was just how big they all were. It was hard not to be in awe of them. They were men whereas I was just a kid. Norman, of course, was playing for Northern Ireland in the World Cup in Spain aged just 17 not long afterwards.

We drew 1-1 and took them back to Anfield, and John said I would be in the squad again. This was big, the biggest game of my fledgling career to date. A match that might attract a crowd of a few thousand.

The night before I'd dug out a pair of Adidas World Cup boots from the pile myself and my brother Jeff used to leave under the stairs at home. I polished them so I could see my face in them. I was determined to look the part. They went into my bag with my shin pads and a towel, everything ready for the next day.

When I reported to Anfield at around 5.30pm, John came over and said I was going to start at centre-forward. Wow – I hadn't been expecting that. I thought I would just be on the bench again. Nerves hit me big time, but I soon had something else to worry about.

I started getting changed. Shirt, shorts, socks, but when it came to putting my boots on something wasn't right. They were really tight.

I loosened the laces a bit and tugged at the sides of one of the boots, to try and widen them and squeeze my foot in. I must have looked like one of the ugly sisters in Cinderella when Prince Charming comes around with the glass slipper. There was no way they were going on.

Then it dawned on me – I'd brought the wrong boots. My brother was a size-and-a-half smaller than me and, in my excitement about playing at Anfield, I'd pulled his out of the pile, polished them up and packed them in my kit bag. His boots. On my big day.

My reaction was fairly predictable: panic. Embarrassment. I could feel my face slowly matching the colour of my red shirt, and I was on the verge of crying. 'This is the biggest opportunity I have had in my career,' I was thinking to myself. 'Imagine going to tell the coach of Liverpool's youth team that I'd brought the wrong boots.' It wasn't the greatest of starts for me.

I think one of the other lads in the team could see something was wrong because, as I became more and more flustered, he asked what the matter was. "I can't find my boots" I said, looking under the bench I was sat on and near to where I was sitting in the changing room. "They were here before."

I was too embarrassed to tell the truth, that I had brought the wrong ones, because I didn't know any of the lads, really. They were older than me and I didn't want them to think the team-mate they would be relying upon to knock Manchester United out of the FA Youth Cup was a half-wit who couldn't manage to bring the right size boots to a game. Eventually, one of them told me to follow him and we went into the boot room near to where the famous 'This is Anfield' sign hangs in the tunnel.

"Just find a pair that fit," he said.

It was a different boot room to the famous one where Shanks, Bob and Joe would sit and talk football with anyone and everyone. Hours spent discussing players and opponents in a little room that played such an important part in shaping Liverpool's history. But that didn't matter to me. I took a pair of Puma King boots, size seven, and headed back into the dressing room for the team-talk, slightly less red-cheeked and with my heart rate having calmed down.

John Bennison was such a nice guy, but he could give it out as well – he wanted to beat United, make no mistake about that. He reminded us of the rivalry between the two clubs and that we were representing Liverpool Football Club. "Don't get too involved though," he said. "Remember what you are good at."

I was aware that Kenny Dalglish wore Puma boots, but if I had taken his boots from the boot room they didn't help me particularly. I had a couple of decent chances in the game. I remember a volley, the ball coming over my shoulder and me snatching at it, with the ball ballooning high and wide into the Anfield Road End. In the second half, when we were attacking the Kop, there was a 50-50 chance with their keeper. I got to the ball fractionally ahead of him, but he managed to get something on my effort and the chance went wide again.

To make matters worse we lost 1-0 and, for a game I was so looking forward to, the feeling at the final whistle was just terrible. I was gutted. I took everything personally. I'd had a couple of decent opportunities and I'd fluffed my lines. I went home worried that, further down the line, people would remember this and hold it against me.

At that stage, I still wasn't sure I would be getting an apprenticeship. St Margaret's was a decent school and, as a result, Liverpool thought I was academically minded and wanted to carry on with my studies, rather than give it all up for a shot at the big time. The situation drifted and drifted. I never spoke about it and they never asked until one day, I felt I had to bring it up. So I approached John.

"We were under the impression you want to stay at school," he said.

"No, that's the last thing that I want to do," I replied. "I want to play for Liverpool."

In truth, my schoolwork had fallen away dramatically as I started to get noticed by teams. From someone who had settled into St Margaret's in Aigburth really well, and in whom the teachers were pleased, my marks had tailed off after the third year as football took over. My mind was always on the football pitch, not in the classroom. Even then, I knew what I wanted to do. But it all hinged upon a club, and Liverpool in particular, being willing to give me my chance.

Thankfully, the impression I had made in Ronnie's impromptu examination of me stuck in the mind of the coaches at Liverpool, longer than my missed opportunities against United. John pulled me aside one day and said I was getting a two-year apprenticeship. No fuss, no fanfare. Here I was stepping out on a path that I hoped would allow me to follow in the footsteps of my heroes, and he was just relaying the good news matter-of-factly.

"See you at pre-season," was basically all he said to me.

I was bursting inside, but not everyone shared my happiness. St Margaret's always had a leavers' service at St Anne's Church, Aigburth, each year for the sixth form and fifth years who decided they were moving on. Everyone's name was read out and, when they came to mine, I could see the head and deputy head do a double take. No sooner had the service ended than I was summoned to see the deputy head, Bob Mander.

I knew what was coming and, sure enough, he said he thought I was making a huge mistake when I said I wanted to pursue a career in football. He urged me to have a rethink. "But that's what I want to do, Sir," I told him, sticking to my guns.

In one respect, it was a compliment that they thought enough of me not to want me to fall by the wayside. In another sense, they obviously didn't think I was good enough as a player. Our school team was poor and, at times, I did wonder if it would hold me back.

I missed one game against Bluecoat because the teachers were so concerned that I was doing so much sport that they asked me to drop out for a couple of weeks. We lost 10-0. When we played them again a few weeks later and I was back in the team, we drew 0-0. I knew I had something, but my conviction didn't seem to be shared by everyone.

Perhaps realising his words had fallen on deaf ears, Mr Mander must have spoken to the headmaster, Robert Naylor, because I hadn't been back in class long before I was summoned to the offices again.

"Do you know how many people attempt that and fail?" the headmaster said when I reiterated my desire to try and make a career for myself in the game I loved.

"I won't. I'm confident I can do it," I shot back. I had belief in what I wanted back then. I may have been quiet, but I was sure I could have a career in football.

4
—

Anfield Apprentice

Liverpool took four of us on in 1982. Paul Leather, Brian Dacey, Tony Tomley and I were all handed apprenticeships and, on our first day, we were assigned the first-team players who we'd look after. Graeme Souness, Craig Johnston, Mark Lawrenson and Phil Neal were on my watch, which meant ensuring their boots were sparkling, their kit sorted and any errands they wanted run being taken care of.

Talk about being thrown in at the deep end. These were some of the best players in Liverpool's history, and some of the most decorated, and it was my job to make sure they had everything they wanted. It felt like a proper responsibility.

It was both exhilarating to be looking after them, but nerve-racking at the same time. I remembered Graeme's spat with Jimmy Case that time at Anfield, and made a mental note to myself to make sure his boots were always gleaming.

Nealy used to give me a pound a week for sorting his stuff out, but if you missed a bit of mud on the bottom of his boots he'd throw them back at you and tell you to do them again. That's just how it was. They constantly tested you to see how you would react. It was all part of growing up and becoming a Liverpool player. It was all to do with respect for others.

The training kit in those days was an absolute disgrace. For starters, it got washed once a week come what may. It was minging. The players had the big woolly jumpers John Bennison had brought for me when he invited me to Melwood as a schoolboy, a V-neck trackie top, a shirt, shorts with no lining, slips and socks. That was it.

One of our jobs would be to bundle the kit together for the players. We'd lay a towel out, put all the kit inside barring one sock, which would be used to tie everything like a parcel, before lugging it away. Actually, in truth, you'd usually just lash it at the apprentice next to you first. There would be bundle fights going on everyday away from the prying eyes of the coaches and first-team players.

As the week wore on, the kit would get heavier and heavier as the players sweated bucketloads. You'd take it down to the drying room and hang it over these wooden rails. They were three rails deep and three high, but the heaters in that room meant that, by the time you came to pick up the kit the next morning, it was like cardboard. You literally had to peel it off the rails, stretch it out and pull it loose.

If Phil Thompson's shorts were black on Tuesday, they still had to last him for the rest of the week. Friday was wash day and that was when it was all sent off to the launderette and a second kit used. It was disgraceful really, and a far cry from nowadays when all the lads have fresh kit every day and there are washing and drying facilities on site.

But they were still great days. I started off being based in the away dressing room. You never went into the home dressing room, unless you absolutely needed to go there. There was no popping your head around the door to see what the first-team squad were up to just out of star-struck curiosity.

"What are you doing in there?" one of the coaches would bark at you. "You've no need to go in there. Get out."

The one excuse you had for poking your head around the door, other than handing the players their kit was if one of them asked you to go on a message for them. Usually it meant an errand to the shops and, more often than not, to the chippy. It wasn't until much later that Liverpool temporarily used the players' lounge at Anfield as a make-shift canteen, and a couple of the girls who worked there laid on some food.

Back then, virtually every lunchtime was spent going to and from the chippy: you'd come back laden with fish and chips, pie and chips, curry and chips, all wrapped up in newspaper, and the best footballers in England would sit in the home dressing room scoffing down their dinner. Imagine that today – Steven Gerrard or Wayne Rooney eating a bag of chips after training. The sports science and nutritionists would go berserk, but it was just par for the course back then and you have to say it didn't do them any harm. I suppose football was less intense in some respects then. There was not the scrutiny Sky television has brought with its ever-expanding grip on the game. I am sure it was similar in dressing rooms up and down the country, but Liverpool stayed ahead of the chasing pack because we had the best players.

Training on a Monday was also a world away from what goes on up and down the country today. Some players would wear a plastic bin-liner under their woolly jumpers to sweat out the alcohol they had consumed over the weekend. Monday was written off, basically. The first team used to play six-a-side matches, but nothing more strenuous than that. Forget your 'Monday Night Football' extravaganzas: back then, it was just accepted that Monday was the day to ease gently back into things, and prepare for the next win.

Liverpool's was a powerful dressing room. Everywhere you looked there were superstars. Apprentices, reserves and the first-team players all used to report to Anfield every morning and then head to Melwood, a few miles down the road, on a bus. We'd mainly be sat at the front and the middle, never at the back, which was where the seniors sat.

Ian Rush and Ronnie Whelan used to get involved with our banter because they were still young themselves. Phil Thompson was another who'd join in. Phil had come through the ranks himself, so he knew how the youngsters felt and tried to put them at ease, offering a word of advice every now and again. He was another of my idols. He was the local lad made good, and quickly became a reference point for every wide-eyed apprentice who was taken on.

But you dreaded Kenny, Graeme or Alan (Hansen) plonking themselves down next to you on the 10-minute trip it took to get to training. Not because they weren't friendly, but simply because you were in awe. I didn't have the confidence to indulge in small talk with Kenny. If he walked on to the bus, I looked elsewhere so I didn't have to make eye contact with him. It was Kenny Dalglish after all. King Kenny.

When Kevin Keegan left, Kenny took Liverpool on to better things. He was just someone who could do everything. He had the touch, the vision, the awareness, and he was tough as well. Bloody tough. People didn't necessarily see that in Kenny. They just saw the wonderful curling shots that would leave a goalkeeper helpless and the inch-perfect passes that would send Rushy sprinting clear. But, if you are not determined and committed as well, all that skill doesn't count for as much. Think of the stick Kenny used to get off defenders and you can see how driven and dedicated he was.

I felt I was making progress, and breaking into the reserves towards the end of my first year as an apprentice was another step forward for me. My debut came on March 15, 1983 at West Brom in the old Central League, and I made my Anfield bow the following month against Bury. Chris Lawler was the manager and I played left midfield. We won 3-0, and I must have done alright because I was in and around the team for the rest of the season.

Whether the games were at home or away, there was a routine the reserve lads got into after a match. The likes of Mark Seagraves, Brian Mooney, David West, Jim Beglin and Kenny De Mange and me would go into town afterwards. Then onto a club – either the Continental or Coconut Grove – have a Chinese meal and then play snooker until about 6am in the old snooker hall in London Road, near the city centre.

That was just the culture. Later on, when I got into the first team, that was the last thing I wanted to do, but back then we followed that routine religiously. We were young, we were doing quite well and the adrenalin was still pumping after a game. Rather than going home and tossing and turning, unable to get to sleep, we'd have a few drinks and relax. Nothing daft: a few bottles of lager, or maybe two or three pints.

Sometimes we'd go straight into training the next day. The staff trusted us and we knew the boundaries. No one was going to jeopardise their career by turning up at Melwood pie-eyed, unable to put their kit on let alone kick a ball straight. Again, it is something that would be frowned upon today. No one was really aware of the effects alcohol has on the body back then, and how it makes you more susceptible to injury. When I was manager of Stockport County I would have taken a dim view of any lads staying up all night. But it just shows how times have changed. Football has become more scientific and focused on how to get the best out of everyone.

Becoming a regular for the reserves so early into my apprenticeship helped my confidence and, after serving my time, I was offered a one-year professional deal. It was worth around £85-a-week, but it wasn't about the money or the length of the contract. Of the four of us who had been taken on together at 16, I was the only one who was retained: the others' dreams had been crushed.

I was gutted for all of them, of course, because we'd had so many laughs, and also scrapes. When Liverpool reached the European Cup final in 1984 against Roma, we went as part of an official club trip. We flew out on the morning of the game and spent the day as a group, walking around Rome and taking in the usual tourist sights like the Trevi fountain, while also mixing with the fans. We also joined in the singing, and generally soaked up the atmosphere.

Basically, you were left to your own devices in the day. You just had to report back to the coach at a certain time, and then you were taken to the game. We had a group of seats reserved by the club and joined in the celebrations when Alan Kennedy continued his knack of scoring massive goals by slotting home the winning penalty against the Italians on their own ground. But our joy was short-lived.

We were dressed in normal clothes – jeans, t-shirt, trainers – and as we were coming out of the stadium there was suddenly commotion to one side of us. It was Roma's Ultras, hell bent on taking some form of revenge on Liverpool. "Leg it," someone shouted.

I heeded the warning, recalling that charge by Chelsea's fans a few years previously, but found myself split up from the rest of the lads because we all just scarpered in different directions. After sprinting for what seemed like ages I found the coach park where we had been dropped, but I couldn't find the coach.

I started thinking: 'What if they've gone without me? What if they've just gone straight to the airport because it wasn't safe to stay here with a mob of Italian lunatics out for blood? What if they don't have a head count and just get as many as they can on?'

It was a panicky time for 10 minutes, running round the coaches trying to see if there was anyone from Liverpool Football Club on board any of them. Thoughts of being stranded in Italy, surrounded by vengeful Roma fans were leaving me in a blind panic. Eventually, thankfully, I found one occupied by some of the lads on the official trip and we pulled away and headed towards the airport. I was safe, at least, and able to dream again about one day maybe helping the club win another European Cup.

Being awarded a professional contract had come as much as a relief, as anything else. The teachers at St Margaret's might just admit they had written me off too quickly now. It was only a deal for 12 months, but that was because the coaches wanted to keep you hungry and ambitious. There could be no resting on your laurels because, if you did, you might be looking for another club within a year. I was happy with that arrangement and felt I was starting to get noticed – and not just by the Liverpool coaching staff.

Nottingham Forest reserves came to Anfield one night. They were always tough to play against and we did well in the game. Everyone was on a high and I walked out of the dressing room and turned right down the corridor, heading towards the main exit when I heard a voice bellowing after me.

"Young man," it boomed. I turned around and Brian Clough was standing at the other end of the corridor in that green baggy tracksuit of his. "Come here," he said, his finger wagging, beckoning me to turn on my heels and walk back down towards him.

"Hello, Mr Clough, how are you?" I said, all polite.

"I am very well. How are you?"

"I'm okay thank you," I replied, thinking it was all a bit surreal that I was having a conversation with Brian Clough, a two-time European Cup-winning manager.

"Let me just say one thing," he went on. "You have a wonderful left foot and don't let anyone tell you otherwise."

Wow. I couldn't believe it. "Thanks very much Mr Clough," I said.

"Now, on your way home," he added, waving me on my way. I think I floated on air as I walked the 20 yards back down the corridor, a smile plastered across my face. This wasn't just anyone giving me praise. It was Brian Clough. 'The' Brian Clough. I couldn't believe it.

No one at Liverpool would have said that. It wasn't their style. Sink or swim was the mantra to them, and handing out accolades did not fit in with that approach. The coaches said "well done" from time to time, but there was never any gushing praise. I burst through the door at home and couldn't wait to tell my dad: "Brian Clough said I've got a wonderful left foot..."

It wasn't the last time Clough's influence would leave a major impression on me. I was 19 when Derby County came to watch me playing for the reserves, after a tip off from Joe Fagan to Arthur Cox and Roy McFarland. I think they had originally come to scout Jim Beglin, but Joe said that he was close to making a breakthrough into the first team and that they should have a look at me instead.

I played and scored twice and, at the end of the game, I was called down to Joe's office. This had never happened to me before, and I didn't know what was awaiting me as I knocked on the door. The boss introduced me to Arthur and Roy and said that they wanted to sign me on loan, and would I be interested in going?

At first I was worried. Was this Liverpool preparing the way to let me down gently and usher me out of the door? Derby were in the old Third Division at the time but, despite my initial concern, Joe explained that he thought it would be good for me to get some experience of playing in a first team in front of proper crowds. I talked it over with mum and dad and, the next day, I got the train down to Derby and stayed in lodgings with Albert and Ruth Standing.

It was the beginning of an adventure I will never forget.

Ruth used to serve up the biggest portions of food you'd seen in your life, so much so that I used to be tempted to push my leftovers into my pockets rather than leave it piled up on my plate so as not to offend her. The football, too, was an absolute education.

Eric Steele, now the Manchester United goalkeeping coach, Kenny Burns and John Robertson, who had both won the European Cup with

Cloughie at Nottingham Forest, were just some of the characters in the dressing room. Those three in particular looked after me. They'd take me everywhere with them. I'd go to the pub, sit down with my half of lager and just listen to all the tales they would tell. So many stories.

John used to come in looking like a bag of shite every morning. He'd have this green bomber jacket on, a cigarette tucked in the back of his hand and he would come in and stand in the middle of the dressing room and recite Clint Eastwood, word for word, from the film 'Dirty Harry'. "I know what you're thinking: 'Did he fire six shots, or only five?' Well, to tell you the truth, in all this excitement, I've kinda lost track myself. But being this is a .44 Magnum, the most powerful hand-gun in the world, and would blow your head clean off, you've got to ask yourself one question: 'Do I feel lucky?' Well, do ya, punk?"

Then he would take another drag on his ciggie. He was absolute class on and off the pitch. What a player.

Kenny was tough as nails and they drove me around, dropped me off whenever I needed to be somewhere, and basically chaperoned me for the time I was there. My debut in senior football came on January 30, 1985, for Derby against Bournemouth at the old Baseball Ground. We lost 3-2, but I really enjoyed my time at Derby. The crowd was good to me. I think they gave me a bit of leeway because I was from Liverpool and so they thought I must have something about me. I would have played a couple more games there but for a hamstring injury I picked up, but I returned to Liverpool buoyed by the whole experience and hoping I could push on – perhaps into the first-team.

There was plenty to look forward to. Everton were winning the title that season, but Liverpool had reached the European Cup final against Juventus and, once again, the club arranged for everyone who wasn't involved with the first team to travel to the game. I can look back at being chased from the Stadio Olimpico in Rome the previous year and smile about it now, but my memories of Heysel still send a chill down my spine. Everything that happened that night was horrific.

We made our own way to the ground that day and our seats in the Main Stand were pretty much right on top of the wall that would later collapse, crushing 39 Juventus fans amid the mayhem and chaos that marred the occasion. You looked at the fencing that segregated the Liverpool supporters from the Italians and thought it was completely inadequate, but you never for one moment considered what was about to unfold. There had been little pockets of fighting, but not to the extent that would have caused a tragedy like that. I thought the police would jump in and sort it out in a minute.

Then I saw the congestion by the side of the wall, the to-ing and fro-ing at the back of the stand, but I still had no real idea as to the scale of what was going to happen until the wall went over and everyone went with it.

Because we were so close to what happened, maybe 30 yards away, some of the sights I saw were horrific. There were tens of people lying on top of each other, others trying to drag them out. While Joe and the team were cocooned away from the tragedy we were sat in among the wives and girlfriends and, like them, saw it all unfold right in front of our eyes. Some of the lads went down below, and at the side of the Main Stand they had started to lay out the dead bodies. There was no escaping the carnage.

The game never should have been played of course, but I suppose the authorities feared there would be more trouble if they postponed the match. We flew home separately from the team that night, but no one spoke on our flight. There was just a stunned hush. Even as young lads, we knew we had witnessed a dark hour in Liverpool's history.

In the aftermath, Kenny took over as manager. Heysel had been such a terrible way for Joe's reign to end, but the appointment of Kenny was an inspired choice by the club. Asking him to be player-manager was an enormous burden at a time when Liverpool were under so much scrutiny, and the ban on English clubs in Europe had just been enforced. How typical of Kenny then, that he should go on to lead the club to the Double in his first season. That success just made me all the more determined to make the step up, although the chance to do so was so very nearly taken away from me.

Hull City, who were managed by Brian Horton, wanted to take me on loan at the start of the 1985/86 season. Garry Parker, who went on to play for Nottingham Forest and Aston Villa, and Richard Jobson, who played for Oldham, Leeds United and Manchester City among others, were there that season and we had a fairly decent side. Again I saw it as a chance to further my experience and I did well there.

I remember speaking years later to Nigel Gleghorn, who had played against me for Ipswich at the old Boothferry Park. "We got the scouting report ahead of that game and it said the left-back doesn't get forward, he sits in position, but he passes the ball nicely," he said. "You never stopped running up and down the flank in that game. I remember going in and saying to the manager: 'Who the fucking hell wrote that scouting report? All I've done is spend the last 45 minutes running towards my own goal.'"

Brian was keen to sign me permanently, and Kenny called me into his office one day.

"There is an opportunity to go if you want to," he said.

My face dropped. Liverpool were telling me I could leave. "No, I think I can play here," I said straight away.

"Fine, no problem," Kenny replied. "You're welcome to stay."

It wasn't a test in the way that Ronnie had set me up when I was still a schoolboy. If I had said 'yes' that would have been it, the end of a dream. I was confident that I was going to achieve my goal of playing for the first team at Liverpool, but I was disappointed that I had been told I could go. I had a point to prove and things I wanted to achieve at Anfield. I was never going to walk away from that voluntarily.

5

Stepping Up

The build-up was just the same as always. I had travelled away with the first team a few times before, but I knew on those early trips that I wasn't going to play unless half the side went down with food poisoning the night before the game. Still, it was a big deal just to wear the club tracksuit, clamber on board the coach to an away ground the day before a match and feel as though you were in and around the seniors.

Whenever one of the young lads got named in a squad, the rest of us used to make a right fuss. Alan Harper went away with the first team for one game and, although the training kit only used to get bundled on a Monday, we made sure his was all properly put together for training before he went on the coach. We also mopped a path from the dressing room door to where he sat in the changing room. We were just messing about really, but that was how much it meant. Being involved with the seniors meant you were getting somewhere.

By December 1986, as I travelled down on the coach for a game at

Charlton Athletic five days before Christmas, I'd already made some subtle signs of progress. Principal among them was the fact that Craig Johnston was my room-mate. From cleaning his boots, now I was sharing a room with him. He was decent to share with, as Craig was quite laidback. There were no constant demands to put the kettle on and make tea for him. The days when I was an errand boy for the best players in England had come to an end.

But, even so, I was still a junior waiting to make his mark. I didn't have great expectations on that trip into the depths of south London. Alan Hansen had been injured the week before, but I still thought I would be the odd one out again.

When we got to Selhurst Park, where Charlton were ground sharing with Crystal Palace at the time, I just filed into the dressing room as normal, merging into the background and staying out of the way as Kenny prepared to name the team. "Bruce, Chico (Steve Nicol), Gaz, Lawro, Jim, Ronnie, Warky, Macca, Giblet (that was me, don't ask me why?!) left midfield..."

Hang on? I looked up, suddenly startled, as Kenny continued naming the side: "...Rushie, Walshy."

This was it. The moment I had waited for all my life. My big chance. And my initial reaction? Fucking panic. I felt sick. Of course I wanted to play and the fact Kenny thought I was ready gave me confidence, but I wasn't prepared. I thought I'd just be warming the bench again.

It was typical of Kenny and Liverpool not to make a fuss about it, and simply reel off my name along with those of the rest of the established lads. Maybe if he had pulled me to one side at the team hotel beforehand and told me that I'd be making my debut, I would have just spent all the time en route to the ground worrying. Now I had no real time to. It was 1.45pm and I had to get changed, warm up and get my head around a position I wasn't totally familiar with. I'd played left midfield before, obviously, but more recently for the reserves I'd been playing left back or even at centre-half.

Later, as I was getting changed, Kenny and Ronnie came up to me and told me to go out and enjoy myself and stick to what I had been doing in training and for the reserves. Enjoy myself? I'm not sure that was what I was thinking. I just wanted to get through the 90 minutes without letting anyone down and blowing my big chance. 'Keep it simple,' I thought. 'Pass and move, pass and move. The Liverpool way. Don't try anything fancy.'

The game itself was a bit of a non-event and ended goalless, instantly forgettable no doubt for most of the 16,564 spectators who had attended, but it will always live long in my memory. Jim Beglin played behind me and helped me through it. I appreciated that. In some respects we were rivals, both looking to play at left-back, but Jim could not have done anything more for me. We knew each other from the reserves so that helped, but he could have left me to get on with things myself. Instead, he made sure I was alright. He was good to me then and has been throughout the illness. Always keeping in touch, always telling me to keep fighting. I didn't do anything particularly brilliant or anything particularly wrong. Just steady, which was fine by me. Charlton would finish fourth bottom, but safe, that season and had some decent players in their side: the likes of Robert Lee, Peter Shirtliff, John Humphrey and Mark Aizlewood. But, even so, Liverpool weren't supposed to draw 0-0 with them. The coach on the way home was fairly quiet. You could sense the disappointment among the players.

So it wouldn't have been right for me to have sat there with a beaming smile on my face, putting my own sense of satisfaction before that of the team. But, inside, I was ready to burst.

There are plenty of lads who had the same dreams as me. Some of those lads were probably more naturally talented than me, but they fell by the wayside for whatever reason. But I had realised a dream. No one could take away the fact that I had played for Liverpool. I sat thinking about that on the five-hour trip home, pinching myself as we crawled back up the country to Merseyside. I had made the step up.

Soon after that goalless draw at Charlton, I came on as a substitute for Paul Walsh towards the end of 3-0 FA Cup second-replay defeat at Luton Town. I had been an unused substitute two days previously in the replay, which had ended in a goalless draw at Anfield, and the schedules meant we played against them again 48 hours later on their plastic pitch. Brian Stein, Mick Harford and Mike Newell did the damage, making our life hell that evening. They gave us the run around on that artificial surface, as they did to so many teams over the years. It's amazing to see how far they've fallen in the years since.

But, after that brief involvement in another inauspicious performance from the first team, I had to wait until April before I was handed another chance to impress. Jim Beglin had broken his leg in a League Cup game against Everton at Goodison Park and Lawro was struggling around that time as well with an Achilles injury. So, with senior figures ruled out, the door swung open again for me to make a mark against Nottingham Forest and my "No1 fan", Brian Clough.

Usually, when you walked into the dressing room on a match day, you knew who was playing straight away. Bruce got changed behind the door and then the shirts were laid out numbers two to five, which was always Ronnie Whelan's jersey, along one wall of the room. On this occasion, I couldn't see around the corner because we turned right when we entered the dressing room, waiting for Kenny to give his team talk. When he said my name, and that I would be playing left-back, three words immediately stuck in my brain: Franz, fucking, Carr.

People might say Franz never quite fulfilled his potential in the game, that his form was always too patchy for someone with his natural skill and pace, and that a player who should have been a world beater ended up more of a journeyman. But, on his day, he could tear any full-back out there apart. I had played against him in the past for the reserves and I was well aware that he could catch pigeons, he was that quick. My introduction to The Kop was not going to be a gentle work out. This was going to be a baptism of fire.

In truth, Forest had a good team back then. As well as Franz, they had Stuart Pearce, Neil Webb, Des Walker, Nigel Clough and Johnny Metgod. They were a test but, although it was my first senior game at Anfield, the nerves didn't hit me as much pre-match. Maybe sitting on the bench, not getting on, against Luton had prepared me in a way for what Anfield was like on match days. I didn't feel like heading for the toilet as soon as Kenny read out the team. Perhaps I'd learned from my brief brushes with the first team that season? I was certainly eager to make a proper, lasting impression this time around.

In the event, I handled Franz quite well on the day, getting tight when I needed to, dropping off when I had to. If the ball was there to be won, I went for it. No holding back. You could get away with more in those days and, while I would never go out to hurt anyone, I did want to make sure Carr would think twice about trying to embarrass me in front of 37,359 fans I was desperate to impress, not to mention my 10 other team-mates and a manager who wouldn't take very kindly to having a weak link exposed in his side.

Yet that was a day, of course, when history would be made and I'd like to think that people remember me for making it... Who am I kidding? Kenny actually played that day and scored what would be his last ever league goal in a Liverpool shirt, and his 172nd since he'd arrived from Celtic for £440,000 a decade earlier. Ronnie Whelan added another and if I had planned how my debut could have gone it would have been like this. I was holding my own and, 2-0 up, even felt comfortable enough to start getting further forward.

It was in the 68th minute when my own moment arrived. The ball had been played into Ian Rush on the right-hand side of the penalty area. He was being shepherded by a Forest defender when he hooked the ball over his head towards the penalty spot where Steve McMahon tried to get on the end of the chance. Instead, one of their players mis-cued a clearance and the ball bounced invitingly in front of me. I had just one thought: to hit it. Thankfully, I caught it sweetly and it flew past Steve Sutton before he could get near to it. Anfield erupted but, while the stadium went berserk all around me and the ball billowed the back of the net, I was there frozen for a split second wondering: 'What do I do now?' My little dose of stage fright – well, sheer embar-rassment, actually – was cured by Steve, who flung himself on top of me before the rest of my team-mates joined in, led by Paul Walsh and Ronnie Whelan burying me at the bottom of a pile of bodies in front of the Anfield Road End. I eventually emerged from a sea of red shirts and trotted back to take up my position, unable to suppress a smile. I felt a weird, tingling sensation, but at the same time it felt amaz-ing. This was another landmark in my desire to prove my doubters wrong. The culmination of four or five years' hard work. Sure, I had played for Liverpool. But now I had scored for Liverpool. At Anfield. With tens of thousands of people clapping and cheering for me. What would the teachers at St Margaret's, who had said I was daft pursuing a career in football, be thinking now?

Back in the changing room, Kenny came over. "Well done," he said, before moving quickly on. That was that. I hadn't been expecting a big fuss. That was the way they did things at Liverpool. Everything was matter-of-fact. We've won, now move on. What's the next game? You're always looking forward, and never back.

Nowadays you might keep the shirt in which you made your home debut, or you'd try and get the match ball you scored with signed by your team-mates, or even your opponents. But there was nothing like that back then. There would have been some funny looks if I'd said: "I'm keeping this shirt for my wall at home." But I did receive one souvenir for my efforts. In return for being voted Man of the Match by the match day sponsors, I received a suit carrier.

Afterwards I headed down to Kelly's on Smithdown Road, a familiar retreat where I knew I wouldn't be bothered. When I was playing in the reserves, myself and all the other lads used to meet there on a Sunday lunchtime and carry on drinking right the way through to last orders. I was never a big drinker, though. I would pace myself, or have a bottle of water in between pints. I was never a person who could drink and drink because I didn't like feeling sick, so I tried never to put myself in that position.

Kelly's was split in two, with a restaurant on one side and a bar on the other. On the night of the Forest game, with the adrenaline still pumping, I just had a meal. There were plenty of congratulations offered by people passing through, and the description of the shot that flew past Sutton got more and more dramatic as the night wore on. In the end, I'd apparently lashed it in from the halfway line and watched it fly into the top corner at 100mph.

There were no big family celebrations. My dad rarely, if ever, went to the games and my mum used to come out in a rash even if she tuned in on television and saw me playing. She couldn't bear to watch, so the thought of visiting Anfield would have filled her with dread, even if I had known in advance that I was going to start the game. It wasn't that they didn't care. They did – passionately. Mum kept a scrapbook of press cuttings during the course of my career, which I still have in a box in the garage somewhere waiting for me to sort out, and my dad always pushed me to do well.

From playing in the school team to the Liverpool senior side, my dad had always been my biggest critic. He'd stand on the sidelines when I was small shouting at me, imploring me to do that little bit more, that little bit better. He meant well, but it got to the stage where I would be shouting back at him. We'd look a right pair, father and son balling at each other while the game went on around us. "Unless you're angry, you never play to your potential," he used to say to me. Maybe he had a point. He was still involved with coaching and managing the police side on Saturday afternoons as well at the time, so if he had come to watch me it would have meant letting them down.

It would have been nice for them to have been in the players' lounge afterwards and to share that afternoon with me, but I hoped there would be more to come. Plenty of other times when I'd be caught in the spotlight. Having said that, you never took anything for granted at Liverpool. This was the most successful team in England, after all, and, until the European ban imposed after Heysel, one of Europe's top teams as well. If they wanted to go out and buy a player, they would go out and buy one. It was only six months earlier that I had had a conversation with Kenny about possibly leaving and going to Hull permanently. I also didn't know whether Mark Lawrenson would recover from his injury, or Jim Beglin from his. I could be back down the pecking order again soon enough.

As pressurised as that made life, there was never any danger of standing still in that environment, and that ensured that your standards could never slip. But, at the same time, this felt good. The games got bigger and the stakes increasingly higher. A few days after the Forest fixture, I started at Old Trafford against Manchester United – we lost 1-0 to a late Peter Davenport goal – and then came the Merseyside derby with Everton at Anfield.

I tried not to get caught up much in the rivalry in the build-up to that game because I was more concerned with going out and proving I could play against the likes of England's Trevor Steven and Peter Reid, or Scotland's Graeme Sharp. The 'Liverpool Echo' would run the build-up to the game all week, whipping the supporters from both sides into a frenzy, although you didn't need the local paper reminding you what was at stake. Training was always sharper in the days immediately before the derby, and just being around players like Steve

McMahon and Rushie, you could tell they were desperate not to lose this game. This game meant everything to them. That much was made very, very obvious.

I wore the number seven shirt that day, though I had enough to worry about without contemplating too much about the significance of a jersey made famous by Kevin Keegan and then Kenny himself. Looking back, it's something else no one can ever take away from me.

Everton had a great team and were on the way to winning the championship that year. Steve scored an absolute screamer nine minutes in, before Kevin Sheedy levelled soon after with a free-kick in front of the Kop. The tension cranked up another notch or two when he flicked the V-sign at our supporters while celebrating, but we hit back again. I managed to provide the crosses from which Rushie grabbed a brace. One of them had Neville Southall in two minds, and Rushie did the rest. It was his last season at the club before his ill-fated move to Juventus, and he was at his best back then. I was simply starting out on my own career, but I was still pinching myself. Having scored on my full home debut, I had now played a big part in a victory over Everton. I felt as if I was making big strides towards winning the supporters over. Maybe I did, really, belong in this company.

Off the pitch, I was getting recognised more and more, although I was never one for walking around wanting to be noticed. That said, I was pretty much on my own. It is a regret now that I never kept in touch with anyone from the school I left at 16. I'd loved cricket as a kid as well and played twice a week for Aigburth during the summer when there was no football, until I decided I had to pick one or the other. I never kept in touch with anyone from the club, either. I don't know whether that shows a focus or determination to do well, or a downright stubbornness on my part, that I allowed both situations to drift as they did. I had good friends at school and good friends at the cricket club and to just forget them... well, I can't say I like myself for doing that. It wasn't intentional. I was simply caught up in trying to forge a success-ful career for myself.

Since I have been ill, I have had cards from Canada and Florida from people claiming to be old boys from St Margaret's, either from my class or the year above, expressing their hope that I was okay and urging me to keep battling. But I've not had a clue who any of them are. Not a clue. I've written back or emailed everyone, but it is a regret now that I didn't pay closer attention to those relationships. There was no reason why they should have just been broken off. But, at the time, I didn't think anything of it. I was in my own little world: one week Anfield, the next at Old Trafford, and then the Merseyside derby to follow. This was what I had wanted all my life.

I didn't even really share those achievements, and my sense of thrill and satisfaction, with the lads I had grown up with at Liverpool, either, because they didn't want to hear how well I was doing. Some of them were still trying to make their own way in the game and the last thing they needed to hear was me saying how everything was going so well for me. And so I kind of told myself I could cope with everything on my own. Or so I thought.

We travelled down to Coventry the week after the Everton win and I was still wearing the number seven shirt, expecting everything to con-tinue going well, blissfully unaware that a reality check was coming my way. During the first half at Highfield Road, I went over awkwardly and was left splayed out on the turf in agony. I thought I had broken my leg and could play no further part in the game, with John Aldridge coming on to replace me. The pain was excruciating, ripping up my leg from just above my right ankle. Roy and Ronnie strapped it up and I sat on the coach on the way home with my leg across the seats, trying to keep the limb elevated. Roy and Ronnie kept coming down the bus to see how I was. They said the sign of a break was a small lump emerging by the impact injury and, after examining my leg, they thought my worst fears would be confirmed.

We got back to Liverpool and Roy took me to Walton Hospital for X-rays. The tests actually revealed there was no break, just ligament damage, much to my relief. I consoled myself in the thought that there were only a couple of games left in the season, so it was not as if someone else could come in and really take my place. Sure, they'd have a little chance to impress, but I'd have a rest over the summer and come back for pre-season ready to push on again, adding to the handful of games I'd already played to become a regular starter for the first team.

But this was my first taste of life as one of the walking wounded. I reported to Melwood on the Monday as usual, and was basically left to my own devices. The staff didn't talk to you if you were injured because you were no good to them. It all went back to Bill Shankly's philosophy. You needed to be available to be noticed. To be considered "useful". So I would go down on the bus to training, sit there and read the paper, have a cup of tea and wait for them all to finish their session.

There was a small multi-gym at Melwood, and you were encouraged to use it or take on a weights programme. That at least kept me occupied for a while, but it was a world away from being out on the pitches getting stuck in during training. I'd eventually catch the bus back to Anfield and, maybe, get put on an ice machine. But it was pretty basic stuff, particularly when you consider the scientific techniques adopted by clubs these days where nothing is left to chance and the attention to detail is enormous. But that was just the way it was back then. Ronnie and Roy would check on you once they had finished their duties with the first team, but that was it.

The trouble was that, by the time pre-season arrived ahead of the 1987/88 campaign, I still wasn't right. The ankle ached and I was dispatched to Park House in Crosby to see a surgeon. It ended up being the first operation I had in my career. The doctors knocked me out and manipulated the joint. When I came round, they said that one of the ligaments had been catching on something and, when it came loose, it had made the sound of a pistol shot. But that wasn't the worst of it. Lying on a hospital bed while my team-mates were out training was not how I had hoped to start a season in which Liverpool were intent upon reclaiming the league title from Everton, and re-establishing themselves on top of the pile. The previous year may have been memorable for me on a personal level, but Liverpool might have considered it a season to forget. They'd even lost the League Cup final 2-1 to Arsenal, with Charlie Nicholas scoring twice. By Liverpool's high standards, it had been a disaster.

While I was in Park House recuperating after the operation, Kenny had turned up with John Barnes and Peter Beardsley to oversee part of their medicals prior to moving to Anfield. They wouldn't have known who I was, particularly, but we were all introduced neverthe-less. Barnesy had been signed for £900,000 from Watford, and Peter for a British record £1.9m from Newcastle United and, as they left, I remember wondering who else Kenny was attempting to bring in. If he had concerns over the fitness of Jim Beglin and Mark Lawrenson, would he be buying a left-back?

My injury could actually not have come at a worse time. I knew then that, despite my run of games the previous season, I would be starting all over again in the months to come. But what if I found myself even further down the pecking order than I had envisaged? Would there be a way back into the first team?

6

—

Fear And Excitement

By the time I was fit again to feature, I found I had a new challenge: myself. When I look back on my Liverpool career, I think it was governed by two contrasting emotions. There was fear and also excitement and it soon became a battle to try and ensure that one outweighed the other. There was the fear of being accepted in a powerful dressing room and of proving myself worthy of a place in Liverpool's first team again versus the excitement of being at such a great club with such an illustrious history. A club I knew I was lucky to be part of.

Sitting in the dressing room, I would look around at all these world-class players – a pool of talent that now included Barnes, Beardsley and John Aldridge, who had joined the previous season – and would wonder what the hell I was doing in there. My ambition had always been to play for Liverpool, and I was well along the path to realising that. I'd come so much further than so, so many of my peers, who had once held the same ambitions. But there was something about sitting in on conversations with the likes of Barnesy that didn't feel right to me. Was I worthy of being in their company?

Just as I had when I'd been lying in a hospital bed with my ankle strapped up at Park House, I'd linger forever on the negatives. I could have thought: 'Well, Kenny chucked me into his team as a 21-year-old and stuck by me, so he must rate me.' But I didn't. I never looked at it that way, taking the positives and pushing any doubts to the back of my mind. Instead, I'd stew in my insecurities. My misgivings were forever threatening my dreams.

I was the one walking down the steps at Anfield, or whatever ground we were at, worrying about not playing well instead of thinking that I would be the best player on the pitch that day. There was a fear factor for me involved in playing for Liverpool because of the pressure that came with pulling on the shirt of one of the biggest clubs in the world. My insecurities held me back. Certainly, these days, the experts might have recognised that here was something to work on, building me up perhaps and eradicating what people would point to as "a lack of mental strength". But it was never spotted, and help never came my way.

I don't know whether Liverpool saw it as a sign of weakness at that time. They probably did. They didn't need to delve into psychology and things like that in the way that clubs do now. I suppose no clubs really did back then, but I couldn't imagine pulling Ronnie Moran to one side and asking him to talk through my problems with me. The staff probably thought that if you needed psychological help, you weren't the right player for them. It went back to the mental test Ronnie would give the youngsters. Sink or swim. Only the strong survive. It was a pretty simple outlook, really.

And so, during the time I played for the first team, I always felt I was very much left to my own devices. There was no difference in how you were treated, regardless of who you were. John Barnes, Gary Ablett, Alan Hansen: your kit was bundled, you trained and you turned up

– as instructed – on a Saturday. I wonder how much better I could have been with some help, an arm around the shoulder, with someone maybe encouraging me to adopt a more positive frame of mind? They could have urged me to believe in myself. They could have convinced me that I was, indeed, fit enough to play and thrive in this company. Could I have been a better player? I don't know. But it certainly would not have done any harm and it might, just, have coaxed something extra from me.

I can't say that I played in the wrong era because, when you look at the success Liverpool enjoyed in the late 1980s – with First Division titles and FA Cup final appearances and successes – it was a golden period. But when you look at the game today, the players have everything. They have psychologists and sports scientists scrutinising how best to eke more from your game, and everyone is much more open to that side of things. In contrast, we had Ronnie and Roy putting you on the medical machines of a morning and lunchtime if you needed treatment. There was no one particularly qualified as far as I could see until Paul Chadwick came in as club doctor later on. But that was Liverpool. That was how we did things. It was like it or lump it, basically.

At my age back then, I wasn't the type of person to turn around and challenge what Liverpool had been doing for so long, and what made them so successful. Instead, I kept my thoughts to myself and, indeed, myself to myself, which may have been a mistake.

I never wanted to be part of the perceived cliques in the dressing room. Rushie, other than for the year he was at Juventus, Ronnie Whelan and Steve McMahon were close. So were the Scottish lads, Alan Hansen and Stevie Nicol. I would keep my own company, and I think some of the other lads took umbrage with that. When they wanted to go out on the ale together, I wasn't particularly bothered. I could take it or leave it and I would say, the majority of the time, I wouldn't go. Times had changed for me since I'd been playing for the reserves and we'd all go out together after games: Continental club, Chinese meal, snooker.

For starters, I had grown up and spent two or three years with those lads, and shared my dreams with them. We were all in the same boat back then. But my team-mates now were lads who were four or five years older than me, and I didn't have that much in common with any of them other than one thing: we all wanted Liverpool to win.

I was happy on my own and I wanted to be myself, rather than be a sheep. Because I was in the team, I didn't feel I needed to do what everyone was asking me to do, or wanted me to do. If I was in the team, playing for Liverpool, then surely it didn't matter if I went out for a pint or not? But maybe I should have made more of an effort. Looking back, perhaps my approach was to my detriment, but the truth was I wanted to be my own man. If I wanted to come in and train and then go home, that's what I would do. If I wanted to come in and train and the lads were going for a drink and I fancied joining them, that's what I would do. It was down to me and what I wanted to do.

Ronnie had a pub called The Sportsman in Kirkdale, a few miles from Anfield, so we always had somewhere to go, somewhere a bit private where we wouldn't be bothered and the invitation was always open. To be fair, the lads could have stopped inviting me, fed up with me knocking them back time after time, but they didn't. I thought I was accomplishing what I set out to achieve and I suppose, from the outside, people thought the same. But supporters only see what goes on of a Saturday, the level of performance and result. The football side, with its obvious highs and lows, never disappointed, but I felt life off the pitch wasn't quite as enjoyable as I'd envisaged. What I was expecting, I don't really know. But I was feeling more and more isolated. I didn't want to feel pressured into going out, so I railed against it.

On the surface, things should have been straightforward that season. After recovering from injury, I played enough league games – 17 – to collect a championship winner's medal in 1988, and was lucky enough to play in one of the most attractive teams Liverpool has ever seen. We didn't lose a game in the league until we faced the reigning champions, Everton, on 29 March at Goodison Park, when Wayne Clarke scored the only goal to end our 29-game unbeaten start to the season.

But that was an exception to the norm. The performances we put on peaked when we demolished Nottingham Forest 5-0 at Anfield. Sir Tom Finney called it "one of the finest displays of football played at pace I've ever seen", and we did indeed hit the heights that night.

As a defender, I didn't have that much to do. We used to give John Barnes the ball and let him get on with it. He would keep it, weave his magic and terrorise opponents week in, week out. Later in my career, I was lucky enough to play alongside a young Paul Gascoigne as an over-age player for the England Under-21s, and his vision and ability to pick out a pass were incredible. But playing alongside John that season was something else. He was just out of this world. He was a magician who used to get kicked from pillar to post or suffer the worst abuse imaginable on and off the pitch, and yet he was someone who just ensured he would have the final say.

Kenny and his staff knew how influential Barnesy was that season and would be in the years to come, but Ronnie would always stick up for the likes of me and Ronnie Whelan. He called us "the ham and eggers", which basically meant we did a lot of the stuff that didn't get any headlines, but which allowed the team to function as one.

My championship medals are in an orange box in the loft, along with my FA Cup and Charity Shield medals.

They're not on show in the house, and I don't get them out very often. Memories are great but the situation I have found myself in since falling ill, I prefer to look forward.

What has happened has happened, I have got my recollections and the odd DVD which I can put on if ever I fancy reliving that period.

That is not to say I don't appreciate it.

Nothing could have made me prouder than doing what I was doing and being afforded the chance to represent that team, arguably one of the greatest teams Liverpool has ever had. It was just unfortunate that we were denied the opportunity to play on a European stage because of Heysel and really test ourselves against the best. I have a fair idea of how we would have done.

When you look at the team we had then, there was Big Al at the back, Steve Nicol, the wizardry of Houghton and Barnes on the wings, the industry of McMahon, the calming presence of Whelan sitting in front of the defence, getting it and playing, tackling anything that moved.

Then you had the out and out impudence and individuality of Beardsley, dropping into holes. The ball that he feeds through the eye of a needle to Aldridge in the first half of the 5-0 win against Forest is well worth watching if you ever get the chance. Simply phenomenal.

And, of course, every time the ball was in the box, Aldo was there to finish it. What a terrible habit to have?! Nothing in football is perfect, but this was near to it.

Being part of that team helped me gain international recognition. The likes of Stuart Pearce and Tony Dorigo were way ahead of me in the pecking order, but I did play for the U21s in April 1988 – and it proved a significant game in the history of English football.

I was called up as an over-age player due to injuries for a European Championship second leg game against France at Highbury. It ended up raining for several hours beforehand and a postponement was on the cards for a while, but the elements didn't prevent me from making my international bow.

England had a decent team then. Perry Suckling was in goal, Martin Keown, Franz Carr and David Rocastle were among the others that played, along with Paul Gascoigne. Yet it was a French forward called Cantona who made the biggest impression. Eric scored twice in a 2-2 draw – we went out because they had won the first leg 4-2 – but more than that, it alerted a host of scouts to his talents.

John Barnes was arguably the best attacking player I ever played with, but Gazza wasn't far behind. I went out with him one afternoon and some of the others while I was with the squad, and we played a few frames of snooker. He was off the wall, just hyperactive and unable to settle. He had to be doing something all the time. But what a player. He could do anything with a ball at his feet. Fantastic.

In December 1990 I featured in an England B game against Algeria. Ian Wright also played and the game finished 0-0. My international career did not last long, but I enjoyed having a taste of it.

Those were good times and were an extension of how it was going for me at Liverpool. We were on the way to winning the league in 1988 and had made it through to the FA Cup final again, with Kenny hoping to win his second Double in three years. What was there that could possibly knock how I was feeling?

Times were good.

Inevitably, the downer came off the field.

When Craig Johnston wrote the 'Anfield Rap' in the build-up to the Cup final against Wimbledon, he based the song around Aldo and Steve McMahon.

'Alright Aldo

Sound as a pound

I'm cushty la, but there's nothing down

The rest of the lads ain't got it sussed

We'll have to learn 'em to talk like us.'

It may sound petty, or even ridiculous, but I took offence at that because there weren't two Scousers in the team – there were three. It wasn't just John Aldridge and Steve McMahon – I was there as well, even if I wasn't as big a name or, indeed, as much of a regular in the team as them. In fairness, from the fourth round of the FA Cup that year, I'd played every game en route to Wembley. But Craig, who had been my room-mate on away trips sometimes, had only written about the two of them so, when it came to shooting the video in Lark Lane one afternoon, there was no way I was going to attend. I didn't want anything to do with it. My view was that if Craig couldn't be bothered to include me in the song, I wasn't going to waste my time helping him with the video. Sure, it seems daft now, but it wound me up at the time.

Again, I didn't say a word. I wasn't the type of person to be confrontational about something like that, and tell Craig how I was feeling and that he should have included me in things. I just stewed on it, bottling it up. It was the same on the nights when we did go out. I knew I'd get hammered for leaving early, branded a lightweight by my team-mates, so I used to go to the toilet and make for the exit afterwards without saying goodbye. I'd escape. I thought: 'Why not? No one is going to remember at training tomorrow anyway because they're all drunk, so I'll get off now rather than put up with the inevitable boring jibes.'

But the video shoot was different. The day after the 'Anfield Rap' had been filmed, we were travelling to an away game on the coach and Big Al got on and started handing the money out: £250 to Barnesy, £250 to Aldo, £250 to Steve McMahon, £250 to Stevie Nicol. Then he got to me. As he handed me the money from the video shoot I had opted against attending, Hansen said: "Listen, you can have the money, but you have got to take part in stuff."

Looking back, I probably shouldn't have accepted it. It is hard when Alan Hansen looks you in the face and puts it right on your toes like he did that day. He was the team captain. I knew he and Kenny were tight, and I knew he was only trying to help me out. I knew he had my best interests at heart. This was some friendly advice I had to take on board.

The thing was that, if I'd explained why I'd not wanted to be involved the day before, the stick I would have got from the rest of the

THE GAME OF MY LIFE

lads would have been fearful. I knew after Alan had spoken to me that this was a situation that could, eventually, count against me but, at the time, it didn't really alter my view of how I should conduct myself. I often wonder now how things might have turned out had I toed the line more back then, being "one of the lads" as they all wanted me to be. Would it have helped my football? I don't know.

What I do know is the distance I kept between me and the rest always boiled down to the mental side of things, to an insecurity and a lack of self-confidence. I'd only ever really gone into the first-team dressing room occasionally back when I'd been an apprentice, and it was rare for me to sit down and just chat with the senior lads. It just wasn't done by any of the younger lads. I never really lost that 'them and us' feeling. I never allowed myself to feel as if I belonged.

I think other people will turn around and say that my attitude was influenced because I was under pressure from my first wife, Debbie. She was a town girl and knew a lot of people. I don't think that went down well with everyone.

The 'Anfield Rap' eventually reached No.3 in the charts, and did decidedly better than we did at Wembley in the FA Cup final itself. No one at Liverpool is allowed to forget the 1988 final. All the stuff Wimbledon came out with about psyching us out in the tunnel prior to kick-off was a load of old bollocks. You are talking about a group of players wearing Liverpool shirts, the majority of whom had confronted the biggest teams in the world, in the biggest stadiums, in front of some of the most ferocious crowds. As if they were going to be put off by Vinnie Jones, Dennis Wise and John Fashanu. No chance.

Wimbledon did make a lot of noise and they were clearly up for the game, but they made noise at Plough Lane, too. That's just what they did. The fact is that we didn't play on the day and, even then, if the referee Brian Hill hadn't disallowed a goal from Peter Beardsley before they scored, it all could have been very different.

I blamed myself for Lawrie Sanchez's header that provided the afternoon's only goal. I should have been tighter. If I had, I might have been able to get my head to the ball first. I didn't, and my mistake was delivered in one of the biggest games of the year. Even then, I still think we thought we would score, eventually. But they doubled up on Barnesy with Wise and Clive Goodyear, and we couldn't get going. Aldo missed the penalty and it wasn't our day.

The dressing room was very quiet afterwards. We knew we had let ourselves down and had ended up on the receiving end of a massive upset that was supposed to encapsulate the romance of the FA Cup. I kept myself to myself, surprise surprise. I'm not one for holding my hand up and saying: "That was my fault." I think that is an absolute waste of time. Everyone knew what had happened that day and looking for scapegoats after the final whistle wasn't going to change the result. In fact, I'd actually recovered in the game to do quite well. I know some people have said I was one of our better players that afternoon, though that is hardly an accolade.

My ability to stay buoyed that day feels more surprising because there were other games – far less important matches – where I would worry about things that weren't my fault in the slightest. For example, I might allow an opponent to come inside and he'd find a team-mate. Three or four passes later, a cross would come in from the other side of the pitch and we'd concede a goal. I would be thinking that it was all my fault. I'd shown him on the inside when, if I'd shown him the outside, I might have conjured a tackle or the move would have gone up a cul-de-sac. Never mind that 20 or 30 seconds had elapsed since my involvement, and that four or five of my team-mates had also been unable to stop the attack. I always put it down as my fault.

It is only now, looking back, that I can acknowledge that wasn't the case and that I was just being far too harsh on myself. In any given 90 minutes, I was obviously going to make a number of mistakes, but I just hoped they wouldn't lead to anything resulting in a goal against us. That is just how the pressure of playing for one of the biggest clubs in the country at the time affected me.

Pretty much everyone else in that team was sure of himself. But I was the local lad and, all the time, I felt I was under greater pressure to go out and prove to the staff, my team-mates and the crowd that I was worth my place in the side. As a local lad, you got the rough end of the stick most of the time. The fans were not going to pick on John Barnes or Peter Beardsley. They were going to pick on an easy target. As much as the fans will turn around and say the lad who came through the ranks is "one of us", you are the first they will turn on when things aren't going well. I was always aware of that much. It nagged at me, played constantly on my mind. There was no escaping it.

Perhaps that's why I don't think I ever truly felt part of things. I played 147 games in five years for Liverpool. But the reality, and the biggest regret, is that I will always feel that I could have done better.

7

Walk On

I pulled on a Liverpool shirt 49 times in the 1988/89 season, the most I ever played for the club in any single campaign. It should be a year upon which I look back with a great deal of personal satisfaction. Instead, whenever I do, the overriding emotion that grips me is actually one of intense sadness.

Over the past 16 months, I have been in and out of hospitals and spent more time hooked up to machines and attached to tubes than I would care to remember. But visiting the victims of the Hillsborough tragedy in a Sheffield hospital is still the hardest thing I have ever had to do in my life. In fact, it was the most harrowing thing any of the lads have ever had to do.

When I turn up for treatment at The Christie, I know what is waiting in store for me. I know the nurses, the doctors, even the treatment I am going to receive. Okay, with cancer, you never really know what is lying around the corner, but I have got my head around that now and

I'd like to think that, whatever happens, I can deal with it.

But when you walk into a hospital unit and a Liverpool fan is lying in a coma with his mum and dad and family helpless at his or her bedside, it is just horrendous. Nightmarish. Even after everything I have been through, there is still no comprehending the pain and the suffering that the victims and their families went through that day in south Yorkshire and, just as significantly, are still going through even now, all these years on.

When you are listening to someone telling you they had hold of a friend's hand, only for them to be sucked away, ripped out of their grasp and lost in a mass of heaving, gasping bodies, what can you say? We listened to their stories in a state of disbelief. Big Al was sick in the corner of one room. It left you numbed. Shocked. Appalled.

One of the parents of one boy asked who had worn the number two shirt that afternoon.

"That was me," I said.

"You are his favourite player."

I was aged 23. Inevitably, it does put my own battle against illness into some kind of perspective.

When we ran out for that FA Cup semi-final with Nottingham Forest, I did think that it was busy behind the goal at the Leppings Lane End of the ground, and wondered why they hadn't delayed the kick-off. So, when we were led back off the pitch at 3.06pm, I wasn't necessarily surprised. I just thought we'd be back out in maybe 10 or 15 minutes once things had been sorted out in the stands.

We stayed in the changing room, shepherded away from the mayhem, with Ronnie and Roy telling us to keep on our toes. Stay focused. Think about the game. If we had known the enormity of the tragedy that was unfolding outside we would have forgotten about defensive drills and how best to hurt Forest, and gone back out to see if we could help – but we were told not to. Instead, the minutes dragged on. Ten, fifteen, twenty. Then there was a commotion at the door of the changing room and a Liverpool fan burst in and shouted out that people were dying out on the terraces.

Silence.

Followed by panic.

My brother, Jeff, was somewhere at the match and I immediately thought of him. 'Was he okay? Was his ticket for that part of the ground?' We didn't have mobile telephones back then, so it was a while before we eventually managed to get in touch. He'd phoned my mum and dad to let them know he was safe and, obviously, I'd made a point of phoning home as well.

I have never really spoken too much about Hillsborough. Not to anybody, and even to my brother. We aren't the closest of families. Jeff has been a policeman for 25 years and he only lives down the road in Great Sankey. If there is a dinner or a family gathering we all get together, but other than that we get on with our own lives, basically. We speak more on the phone now since my illness.

But we're not immune to things, and I'm sure memories of that horrendous afternoon still linger for both Jeff and I. How could you not be affected by what happened that day? I still look back at those events now and upset myself, welling up at the thought of all those fans who went to a football game and didn't come home. There were 96 funerals, of which I attended 11. Whenever I was asked to, I put my name forward. I was a local lad and wanted to help because these were my supporters as well. I was one of them. Whether it was helping to carry a coffin or reading a service in church, which I found incredibly difficult, I tried to do my bit. Not out of a sense of duty, but because I wanted to. This was our tragedy.

Usually I would break down. I'm not ashamed to say that. But everything was so over-powering: the emotions and feelings of that terrible, dark day; the loved ones who had been lost; the ages of those who had died. It was horrendous. All of it.

I only ever kept two Liverpool shirts over my career and one of them I gave to Phil Hammond to put in the coffin of his son, Philip Jnr, who died aged just 14. St Margaret's, where I had gone to school, was just across the road from where Phil lived, and I was asked to attend the funeral. Offering the shirt was just something I thought was the right thing to do.

I can remember, in the days immediately after the tragedy, we walked out at Anfield and saw the wreaths, scarves and flags which were spreading all the way across the pitch, and the tributes on the Kop. A lad came up to me, just dressed in his jeans and trainers, and broke down crying.

"I've got all my savings out of the bank," he said. "Make sure they go into the appeal fund for me." Then he handed me a big wad of cash.

I broke down as well.

That's just my story.

John Aldridge just wanted to walk away from football altogether. This was his club, and these were his supporters who had suffered so much. They were mine as well but, growing up, I probably didn't have the same passion for Liverpool as John. It affected him profoundly.

Then there was Kenny and his wife, Marina, who were legends, absolute legends, for the way they conducted themselves in the immediate aftermath and in the days, weeks, years and decades since. They were virtually locking Anfield up at night because they'd spent the day there, offering a shoulder to cry on for a lot of the relatives who found spending time in Kenny's company a way of coping with their sadness.

There was a time immediately after the tragedy when no one spoke about football. It was an irrelevance. A distraction. But, eventually, we understood what we had to do. The people who had lost their lives had gone to a match and to see us play, and I think it would have been wrong for us not to carry on. We had the memory of those 96 people to play for now.

In the end, our route back into playing again took us up to Celtic Park for a Hillsborough Memorial game. Hearing the bellowed chorus of 'You'll Never Walk Alone' echo around that arena before kick-off and during the game was spine-tingling, hairs on the back of your neck stuff. We won 4-0, with Aldo scoring twice and Rushie and Kenny once each, but the result wasn't important. Rather, it was just a chance to get out, run around and stretch your legs away from the training pitch against different opposition. A chance to get back into what already felt like a distant, old routine.

After the game, Kenny had booked out a restaurant in Glasgow for us all. In a small way, this was our night. A chance for us to let all of the emotions that had built up in us over the previous two weeks come flooding out. It was an opportunity to go out as a group, have some good food together, even have a sing-song and try, as much as you could, to get back to some sense of normality.

Kenny had also arranged through a friend of his, Tony Bruce, for Marti Pellow, the lead singer of 'Wet Wet Wet', to put on a show. We knew Marti because he'd been to Melwood a couple times in the past, and joined in with us sometimes in training. He was a fantastic entertainer and got up and started singing. He'd sung three or four songs and was absolutely top class, but by then we were all full of ale and wanted to take over the mic ourselves.

And who was first up? Me, grabbing centre stage from Marti and belting out Shirley Bassey's 'Big Spender'. It was probably awful. Jacqueline says I've not got a great singing voice, but I think the lads were too shocked to notice how bad I was. Everyone was like: 'What's he doing?' I was meant to be the quiet one, but it was just that type of night. In the end, everyone got up and had a go.

My thinking was that, by taking the bull by the horns and getting it over with, no one would be picking on me and turning my song into a massive thing. Marti? Well he saw his arse and went home early.

After playing Everton in the league at Goodison Park, we resumed the semi-final with Forest. We knew we had to win. Excuses would have been made for us if we had lost, but we didn't want anyone's sympathy. We wanted to get to the final and make sure we made everyone proud of us. We played well at Old Trafford, winning 3-1, and John will always be remembered for rubbing the top of Brian Laws' head after he scored an own goal, something he probably regrets. But it was simply the emotion of the occasion coming out again.

In many respects, the final was just the same although the fact that we were meeting Everton ensured any slip-up was all the more unthinkable. It was a hugely emotional day. The sheer volume of fans who wanted to be there meant, sensibly, some were allowed to sit around the side of the pitch by the authorities.

Nothing was going to stop us that day. We weren't destined to win simply because of what had happened. Everton wanted victory badly themselves, so they weren't going to roll over. Cup finals are cup finals, as we were only too aware, given Wimbledon's triumph the previous year, but I always felt we were the better side.

Graeme Sharp was a handful for any centre-half. He was a strong, clever player and I speak to him a lot now still, but I thought I did well against him that day. Aldo had put us in front early on, but we conceded an equaliser in the last moments of normal time. I was so close to getting a toe on the cross-shot from Pat Nevin that Stuart McCall tucked home with seconds left, but the ball just evaded me. I remember Stevie Nicol getting up and taking a massive swipe at McCall as he ran away in celebration. Other, lesser teams might have panicked at being pegged back like that.

It would have been easy to fold, but when you have players like Rushie and Barnesy around, you know one moment of magic can turn the game back in your favour – and so it proved. Rushie put us back into the lead but McCall equalised again with a breathtaking volley. However, Rushie reigned supreme against Everton, as his record of 25 goals against them in a Liverpool shirt showed, and he invariably managed to have the last word, which he did again with a deft header from Barnesy's pinpoint cross.

I would have loved to have done a proper lap of honour, even in the garish yellow and red bobble hat a supporter had thrown at me and I'd plonked on my head. But, with the fans having been let onto the running track around the pitch at Wembley, it wasn't advisable. We had the usual post-Cup final party in a hotel in London afterwards. Some of the lads could drink all night, but not me. I was tucked up in bed by 1am with my medal on the bedside cabinet.

My medal collection was starting to build up nicely, and I still had eyes on securing one more piece of silverware that season. Our league campaign had been strange that year. We were off the pace – we actually slipped 19 points off the top at one point – and we weren't as consistent as usual. Before one game, Ronnie Moran and Roy Evans had turned to the lads in the dressing room and, pointing to me and Ronnie Whelan, said if it wasn't for the pair of us hauling everyone out of the shit each week, they didn't know where the team would be.

To receive that kind of praise from coaches as shrewd as Ronnie and Roy, and for it to be delivered in front of your team-mates, was tremendous. A really proud moment. And it wasn't said for effect. They meant it, and that's why it stands out in my memory.

Despite a sticky patch by our standards, good teams always recover and find a way to win. We gathered some momentum and went on an unbelievable run, winning 13 games out of 14 (the other was the goalless draw with Everton in the derby after Hillsborough) that took us into the final game of the season against second-placed Arsenal with the destiny of the title in our own hands.

Looking back now, it proved a game too far for us. In my opinion,

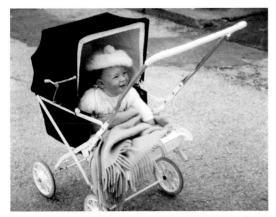

Early days and dressed in blue. But the first team I followed was Liverpool

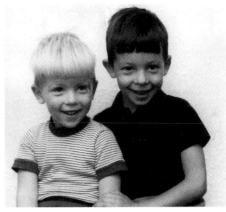

Me and my brother Jeff – I later took his boots to my big trial by mistake

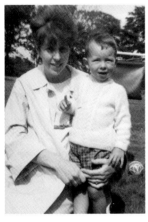

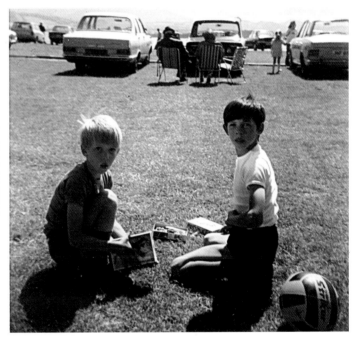

Me in Sefton Park with my mum and (right) on holiday in Beaumaris in North Wales with Jeff again. As you can see from both photos, a ball was never too far from my side

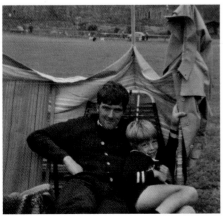

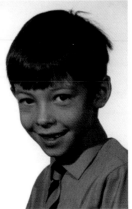

Aged eight and full of dreams, looking smart in my school uniform and (far left) my dad with Jeff. Dad followed my progress closely

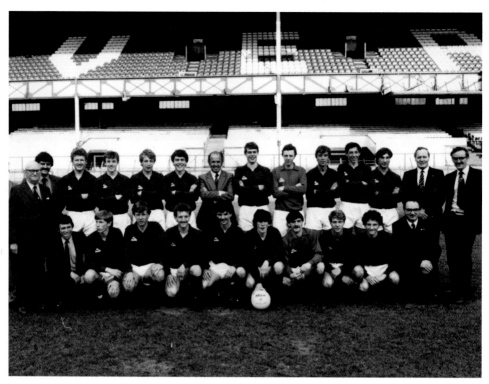

A taste of the big time: Lining up for Merseyside Under-19s at Goodison Park. I'm on the back row, fourth from left. I was aged only 16

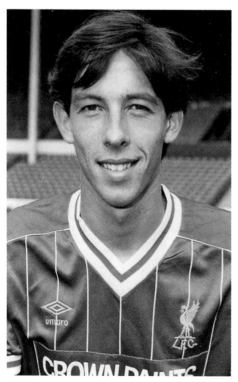

My first pre-season photocall, summer 1984

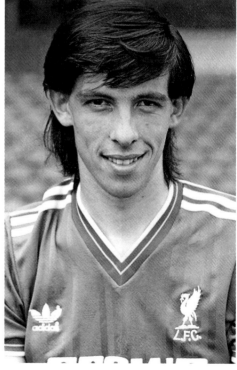

New season, new mullet, pre-season 1985

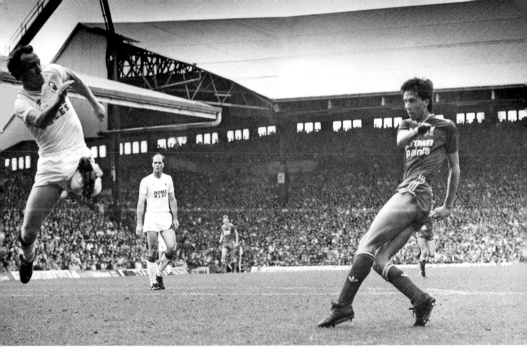

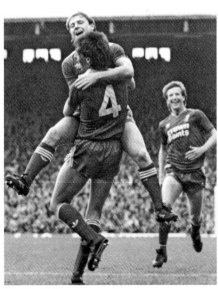

My first – and only – goal for Liverpool 'lashed into the top corner from the half-way line at 100mph'... allegedly!

How do I celebrate? Steve McMahon saves me from my stage fright, left

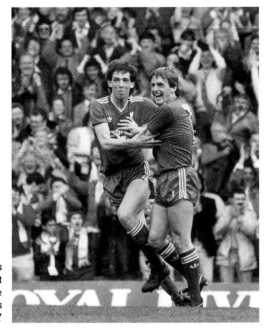

My role model: I always looked up to Kenny. I'm first to congratulate him on one of his many goals in this picture from April, 1987

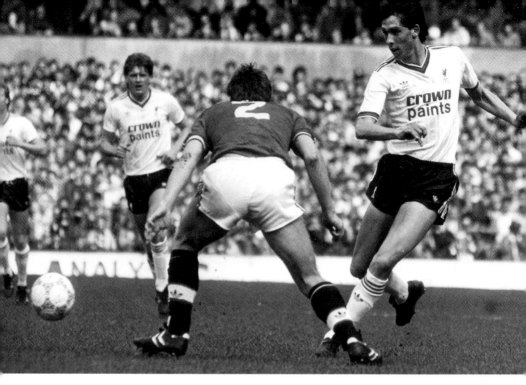

The old enemy: In action at Old Trafford. I might have ended up wearing a United shirt – had they not played me in goal on trial!

My first Merseyside derby day, as Liverpool's new number seven. Far right, the 1988 FA Cup final ... the less said, the better

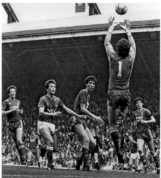

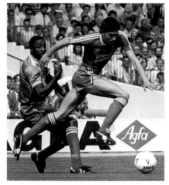

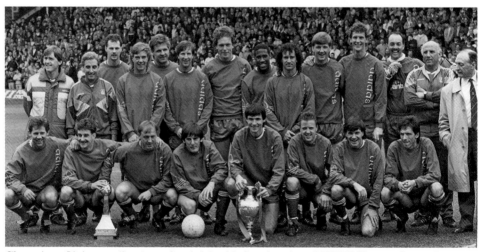

Champions: Lining up (front row, far right) with the victorious 1987/88 Liverpool squad

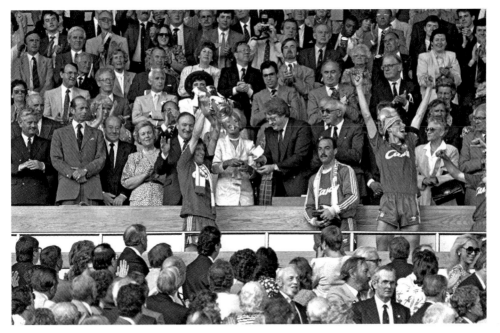

Cup winners: Dodgy bobble hat and arms aloft, as Ronnie Whelan raises the FA Cup in 1989

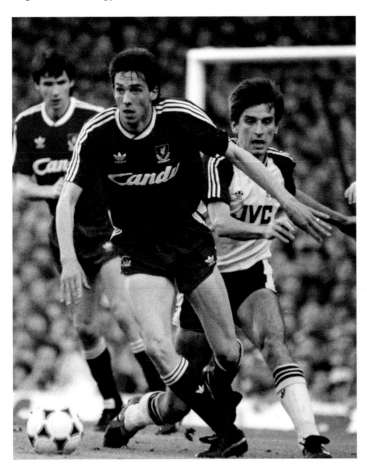

A game too far: Beating Alan Smith to the ball in *that* game against Arsenal in 1989. Smith would end up having the last laugh

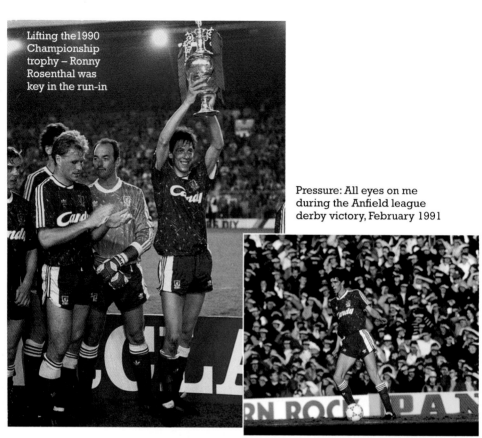

Lifting the 1990 Championship trophy – Ronny Rosenthal was key in the run-in

Pressure: All eyes on me during the Anfield league derby victory, February 1991

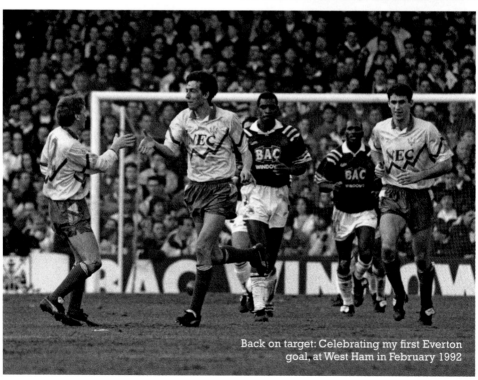

Back on target: Celebrating my first Everton goal, at West Ham in February 1992

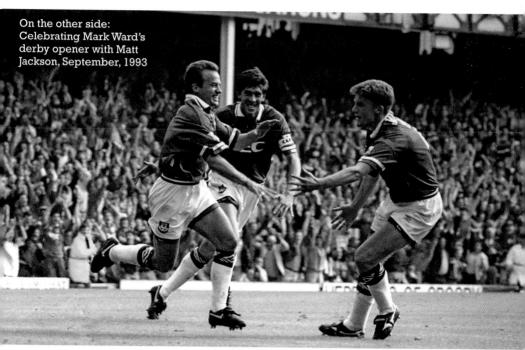

On the other side:
Celebrating Mark Ward's
derby opener with Matt
Jackson, September, 1993

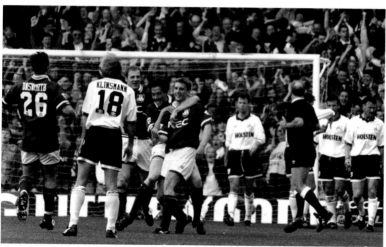

What dream final? I'm first
on the scene following Matt
Jackson's opener in the 1995
FA Cup semi-final victory over
Tottenham Hotspur

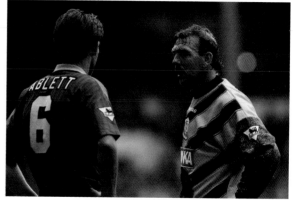

'Just roll the ball to me, Nev,
and give me an early touch'
... in discussion with the one
and only Neville Southall

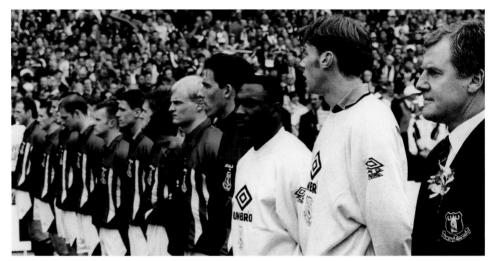

Deep in thought ahead of the 1995 FA Cup final (fourth right), alongside my team-mates

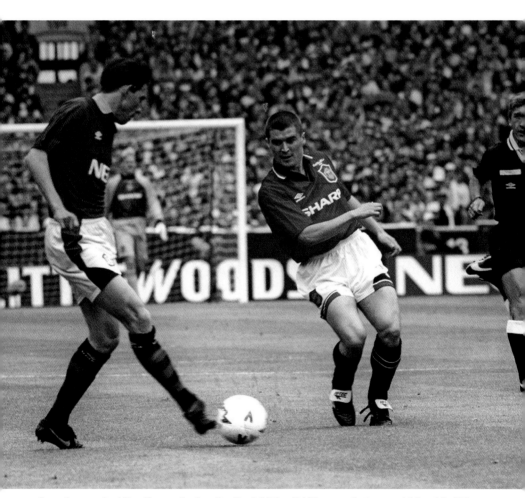

In action against Roy Keane during the final. Little did I know what a good friend he'd become

we didn't know whether to stick or twist, go for the game or sit off Arsenal. George Graham's side had to win by two clear goals at Anfield to wrench the championship from our grasp. We'd only lost once at home all season, and then only narrowly to Newcastle. Surely Arsenal couldn't turn us over by two goals. That couldn't happen, could it?

Liverpool's reputation was carved on our ability to perform in the big games, when the expectations were fierce and the stakes at their highest. But that night we flopped. Alan Smith scored early in the second half to leave us jittery, but everyone recalls the image of Steve McMahon frantically reminding us all that there was only a minute left. Sixty seconds to hang on and complete what would have been the most emotional Double in the history of football. Sixty seconds. It was within our grasp.

I don't need to watch a DVD or video of the final few moments of that season to jog my memory as to what happened next. The move that brought Arsenal victory remains seared on my mind. It always will be. John Lukic rolls it out. The ball is pumped forward by Lee Dixon. There's a flick on by Alan Smith. A touch. A ricochet. And Michael Thomas bursts through the middle and hoists it in the net. Sixty seconds, and then it was gone.

I probably should have been a bit closer to Smith in the build up, but it was the 92nd or 93rd minute and everyone was out on their feet. Full credit to Arsenal. They came and did a job and, while they celebrated on the pitch, receiving a generous ovation from the Kop, we slunk back into the changing room. Beaten. All the champagne was going back in the cases, and Ronnie and Roy wouldn't be handing out medals from the orange box this time around. That Double had gone.

I am a little embarrassed to admit it but, when I sat down in the dressing room trying to make sense of what had gone on, all I was initially thinking about was that Michael Thomas' goal had just cost me £10,000. We had received £5,000 for winning the FA Cup, we would get another £5,000 for winning the League Championship and then there would be a bonus of £5,000 for pulling off the Double. It may seem a pittance when people consider what footballers earn these days, but £10,000 was a lot of money back in 1989. An awful lot.

But, thankfully, a sense of realism did sink in eventually. Losing that game, and with it the title, was a desperate way to end a season no one will ever forget – and nor should we.

For the victims of the Hillsborough disaster, the 96, the fight goes on. The dedication and determination with which they have fought in the years since to ensure the truth comes out is truly inspirational.

Finally, it seems there is a determination among the powers that be that the truth will come out, that someone will be held accountable for what happened. I hope then there will be some sort of closure for the families who lost their loved ones.

8

Getting Stick

The summer brought rest and respite but, going into the new season, ours was simply a sense of unfinished business. There was no sense that things needed to be radically altered. Why should they be? Kenny had come close to winning three trophies in his first season – people forget we lost the League Cup semi-final to Queens Park Rangers, that defeat understandably forgotten amid the glory of the Double that was achieved. We should have claimed a Double again in his third season, only to lose to Wimbledon in the FA Cup final. And then there was the Arsenal defeat in the final minute of the final match that denied us another league and cup clean sweep. But those were near misses. There was no real need to change anything.

Pre-season was the same. The same drills. The same approach. But everyone still had the memory of Michael Thomas' late, late goal imprinted on their minds. Kenny might have changed a bit in the years since in terms of becoming more of a tactician, but back then I think he and his staff just knew that, deep down, they simply had the best players out there. As long as we passed and moved, we would be okay.

It was all about us. The only time we ever thought about changing things around because of who the opposition were was when we played Arsenal at Highbury. Peter Beardsley might miss out because Kenny thought he was too small to make an impression against their defence. But, otherwise, we concentrated on ourselves. Doing things the Liverpool way. Doing what was best for us.

It was the atmosphere around the place that sticks in the memory. We had the same teams in five-a-side for two or three years running: the staff versus the others, and Kenny was always just a joy to watch. Always one touch. Always the right pass. Once again, I was on the staff team and used to play in goal. My job on a Saturday was to hold the fort at the back and try and read the game being played out in front of me, so I didn't mind going in nets for those games. I never moved. It felt as if I had broken wrists from trying to stop shots Jan Molby had battered at me from 10 yards. We'd have Kenny, Roy, Ronnie, Big Al, Steve McMahon, Rushie and some of the other older lads playing for us in the staff side. The opposition never stood a chance.

I think other teams in the league were probably more tactically minded than us, but then they couldn't handle our passing and movement. They call it 'working between the lines' now. Rafa Benitez was always going on about finding the space between the midfield and defence, but it wasn't a new thing. We had Peter doing it back in the late 1980s and early 1990s. He would drop into space and feed players with little balls down the side of the centre-halves for John and Ian to collect. It was years ahead of its time without us even knowing it.

We used to do a lot of time wasting back then. Bruce would roll it out. I would put my foot on it, before sending it back to him. Then he'd roll it to Big Al and he'd put his foot on it for 20 seconds, or until someone came and closed us down. It was just to take the sting out of the game. We could all defend and weren't afraid to put our heads in the way of anything – you only have to see the clash Gary Gillespie and Nigel Spackman suffered against Luton just days before the 1988 FA Cup final to see that – but there wasn't a time when I felt we were consistently put under pressure and where we had to scrap for our lives. So everything stayed the same.

There was a wonderfully familiar routine to it all. In training we did the same stretches, the same shuttles, the same doggies and used the shooting and rebound boards. If there wasn't a game, you knew what you would be doing every Monday, every Tuesday, every Wednesday, every Thursday and then we would get the biscuits out on a Friday morning. There was a little tradition whereby Kenny, or one of the lads, would bring some chocolate digestives down on a Friday and we would have them with a cup of tea before training. Then we couldn't start the session until Bruce had scored past another keeper with an overhead kick. You'd have the lads crossing balls to him and Bruce would be acrobatically flinging himself around, desperately trying to score with a scissor-kick. When the first one missed, he'd drag himself up and try again. It would go on for ages some weeks, depending on his accuracy, and on those occasions the staff would step in.

Eventually, either Ronnie or Roy would lose patience and bark out: "Right, that's it. Enough. We've only got an hour left, so let's get on and do what we have to do."

It used to wind Bruce up when he'd been off target a few times and John Aldridge would step forward and, bam, he'd belt it into the bottom corner from the first cross sent over for him with the goalkeeper nowhere to be seen. The rest of us would break into applause, cheering John, knowing it would be driving Bruce on to try and try again.

Out of all my team-mates, Bruce was undoubtedly the biggest character. Every morning he'd come into the dressing room, get changed and put his eye drops in. But that's pretty much as predictable as he ever got. Once we were sat in the old square baths at Anfield, the water up to our knees, when Bruce comes shinning along the drainpipe that ran across the ceiling, completely naked. He's hanging upside down, 8ft up in the air, and we're thinking: "What the fuck is he up to now?"

Next minute, splash. He just belly-flopped into the water. What is it they say, again? About goalkeepers being mad...

His stories about being in the army were phenomenal. He'd tell you how to kill a snake with your bare hands.

Bruce was a great goalkeeper as well. I thought Neville Southall was better than him and having gone on to play with Neville, I have no reason to change that opinion. But take nothing away from Bruce. As a defender, you knew whenever anything came into the box there was a 75-80 per cent chance that he would come for it. It took the pressure off us enormously. We'd just try and offer him as much protection as we could. Either that, or we'd run back to the goal-line in case he dropped a cross and we had to clear a shot off the line.

Sitting there and listening to the banter that used to go on in the dressing room was an education. Big Al and Stevie Nicol were the worst, a Scottish double act. They would arrive in the morning and Big Al would pipe up: "Did you see that programme on the television last night from Sweden with Bo Bo-son?"

"No," said Stevie. "But I saw the one that was on with Sven Svenson and Anders Anderson."

They would go on and on happily for hours, conjuring up all these different names, and the lads would be creasing up in the dressing room, laughing at their little comic routine.

At times I still felt like I was on the outside while all the banter was going, and I remember an incident with Steve McMahon where I took the opportunity to stand up for myself and tried to earn some respect. There was a fridge full of Lucozade in the dressing room at Anfield and, when we came in to get changed before training, we would have a drink and sit around talking and messing about. Socks would get hurled across the dressing room at each other, trying to catch one of your team-mates unawares.

One morning, Steve was sat about five yards away when he lashed a rolled up sock at me as though he was flinging a ball at a coconut shy on a fairground. Bang. Not surprisingly, my drink went flying out of my hand, Lucozade spilling everywhere and leaving me drenched. For a second I was stunned, but then I realised it was a chance for me to make a point. Okay, I wasn't an accepted member of any of the cliques but, at the same time, don't take the piss.

If the sock comes flying from across the other side of the room, then fair enough. At least you have time to react. But this was like asking Bruce to save one of Barnesy's thunderbolts from point-blank range.

"What the fuck are you doing?" I shouted, my face like thunder.

Steve just laughed, almost nervously, and the moment quickly calmed down, the tension ebbing away, but I think I'd made my point. I wasn't some dickhead who'd take anything lying down. Hopefully, he respected me more as a result of it. Steve is a tough lad and I get on well with him whenever I see him nowadays, which isn't often admittedly given that he lives on the other side of the world. But I wasn't going to be steamrollered, bullied even, by people. I wasn't putting up with that.

Deep down, though, I knew that in that dressing room respect was only earned courtesy of what you did out on the pitch, and I was starting to feel I was justifying myself at this level. My best-ever game for Liverpool came in a 5-2 win at Chelsea in December 1989. I was on fire that day and John Hollins, the former Chelsea manager-turned pundit, praised me to the hilt in a newspaper afterwards, saying that he had never seen a left-back run a game before.

We ran riot at Stamford Bridge that day. Rushie, inevitably, got a couple. Peter scored, while Ray Houghton and Steve McMahon helped themselves to the rest. But it was the left-back who apparently caught the eye. There are some matches when it just happens for you. You get an early touch and, when the ball comes off your foot, it just feels so right. It clicks. Your confidence flows and you feel you can do anything.

Recently I managed to get a DVD showing some highlights of the match because that, for me, was everything I wanted my Liverpool career to be, encapsulated in 90 minutes: a really good win coupled with me playing my part, so that everyone in the dressing room would think 'Abbo did well today', even if they didn't say it out loud.

Goodness knows why, but Kenny clearly thought he couldn't rely on me to play with that same attacking verve every week! A few months later, he went out and signed Ronny Rosenthal from Standard Liege, initially on a loan deal that eventually became a permanent £1.1m transfer. He went on to be nicknamed 'The Scud' as a result of never being on target, like the missiles in the Gulf War that always seemed to be destroying civilian targets, or even hitting our own troops. But, jokes aside, Ronny did well for us and scored the perfect hat-trick against Charlton one night: left foot, right foot and header.

When he was signed there weren't that many people who were aware of him. He was a bit of an unknown quantity and had this really strange running style, like a goblin. But he was very effective. We weren't sure physically whether he would cope in England, but he scored some vital goals and pushed us over the line that season.

Without the impetus Ronny gave us, we might not have won the title. Aldo had left for Real Sociedad in the autumn after the 9-0 win over Crystal Palace, meaning that Ronny was a welcome addition.

That League Championship in 1990 remains, to date, the last claimed by the club. To think now that I am still a member of Liverpool's last championship-winning team is ridiculous, although I've seen the teams since and, collectively, they have never understood the pass and move philosophy that we had. Or, if they have understood it, then they simply haven't had the players to put it into practice effectively. There have been too many bad buys in the years since. Far too many.

Mind you, at the time, if you had said that would be Kenny's last title with Liverpool as well you would have found yourself sectioned. From a selfish point of view, I was sad to see Kenny leave mid-way through the following season. He had given me my chance, handed me a route into the first team and working with him had been a privilege. When I'd told him I didn't want to go to Hull all those years earlier, he could have taken the hump, but he treated me fairly. He was my player-manager, and the man who allowed me to fulfill my dreams. Others may not have offered the same level of support or faith in my ability. He stuck by me and I will forever be thankful to him for that.

It is very difficult to gauge what Kenny had been through in the aftermath of Hillsborough and how the stress had affected both him and his family. He took on so much himself, but he wasn't a counsellor, properly trained in dealing with helping people through this sort of trauma. None of us were.

Kenny said the day he quit was the only time he has ever put himself before Liverpool Football Club, and no one should begrudge him doing that. He just needed to recharge his batteries and have a break.

Really, with the benefit of hindsight, the club should have done more to check on how much Kenny wanted to come back in the months after his resignation before making any hard and fast decisions. They owed Kenny that much at least.

The day he resigned, we were all sat in the dressing room waiting to see what was going on and what would happen next. It was a Friday and we were travelling to Luton. There was a real sense of uncertainty that none of us had ever experienced at the club before. No one really knew what would happen next. That wasn't Liverpool. It was always all mapped out for us. We all knew what we were doing and where we were going. This was different. There was a genuine sense of sadness.

So in walked Al, flanked by Ronnie and Roy, with an announcement to make. "I've just had a meeting with the board of directors," he said. "They have offered me the job of manager."

The reaction was spontaneous, everyone welcoming the news and offering congratulations, but Al hadn't finished.

"Right," he continued, "there are going to be some changes around here. You, Steve Nicol. I know where you drink, and you won't be drinking any more."

Stevie's face dropped.

"On Sundays, you lot will all be in watching the video of the previous day's game. We're going over things with a fine-tooth comb. Things have become sloppy and they are going to change around here. Things are going to change, believe me."

Stunned silence. Oh my God. The thing was, we all knew that if Al was going to make the step up to management, it would have to be done in an instant. You couldn't integrate him into a new role over a period of time, allowing people to take advantage of him. This was credible. Hansen, the boss, was apparently going to rule with an iron rod. No more banter with the boys, no more comedy routines with Stevie. With him as manager, we were going to be whipped into shape.

Al was straight-faced, surveying our flabbergasted reactions. Nicol was speechless. Choked. Ronnie and Roy, at Hansen's side, were just nodding grimly. Then the big man couldn't hold it together any longer and just creased up laughing.

"You bastard," was Stevie's curt response. Ronnie stood in as care-taker-manager, taking up the reins as we attempted to catch Arsenal in the First Division. But, as it happens, I was soon wishing Al had actually taken over pretty soon.

* * * * * * * * * * * * * * * *

When Graeme Souness was appointed as Kenny's permanent successor, my first thought was: 'Thank God I polished his boots properly all those years before.' But I don't think I was ever a Graeme Souness type of player. I wanted to bring the ball down on the floor and try and play football. Graeme wanted me to kick the striker I was marking, which wasn't my natural game.

Don't get me wrong: if the ball was there to be won, I would win it. But being aggressive for the sake of being aggressive, trying to intimidate opponents just to look macho... well, that didn't sit right with me. But, from the start of Graeme's tenure, I just felt that there was an undertone that he wanted us to kick anything that moved.

His first full season back in charge, 1991/92, was the first year we were allowed back into European competition after our ban for the Heysel disaster had lapsed. The opening UEFA Cup tie saw the Finnish part-timers Kuusysi Lahti come to Anfield, a game we won 6-1 with Dean Saunders, recently arrived from Aston Villa, scoring four goals. That huge victory meant narrowly losing the second leg over there was irrelevant.

We played Auxerre in the next round and were staring down the barrel after losing the first leg 2-0 in France. No Liverpool team had ever overturned a two-goal first-leg deficit before but we knew that, if we could get an early goal, the momentum would be with us. It all seemed to hinge on ensuring we scored first and seized the initiative.

Auxerre had a Hungarian forward at the time, Kalman Kovacs, who had scored in France. I remember going through the back of him right on the half-way line. It was a poor challenge from me, one which betrayed my eagerness to play a part in what we hoped could be a famous European night, and he had to limp off. But, with their key forward off in the treatment room recovering from my foul, Auxerre wilted. Jan Molby scored an early penalty, Mike Marsh added a header and then, late on, Mark Walters scored the winner to leave the Kop delirious.

When we got back into the dressing room after the game, Graeme came over to me. "Well done, great tackle," is all he said. But I knew it wasn't a great tackle. I'd mistimed it, but it was clear that is what he wanted. None of it sat easily with me.

Soon afterwards, the lads all went out together to the Sportsman and, for once, I tagged along. Everyone was there, other than Souness, and I ended up speaking with Roy Evans in a corner. You could always talk to Roy. He was like an official minder for the lads in that environment and, while we were chatting over a drink, the conversation drifted on to the Auxerre match. "That's not your game, is it?" said Roy.

"That will never be my game, going around kicking people."

My intention was always to go for the ball. I might mis-time challenges now and again, like I had that night, but I would never go out there with the intention of hurting anyone. At no point in my career was that my motivation. I'm not daft enough to think you can win the ball fairly every time. There are occasions when you have to commit a foul, and there were times over my career when I was sent off for poor challenges. But, on the whole, as a professional footballer my game was about trying to win the ball, to read the game and to give it to the lads who could play. If I achieved that, I could spend my time organising things behind them: who we pick up, who goes towards the ball, who picks up who. It was hardly the 'enforcing' role Graeme clearly wanted me to play.

But I wasn't alone in wondering if I fitted in under the new manager. Big Al was on his way out with his knee problems starting to limit the impact he could make. Neither Steve Nicol nor Gary Gillespie were comfortable, either, playing that way. Things were changing. Overall, Graeme's style of management was overly confrontational, which wasn't my cup of tea. It soon became apparent that I wasn't his, either.

I found myself being moved around the team to accommodate other players, and I even ended up playing left midfield in some games, a position I had not played regularly for years. It just made me wonder what the hell was going on. I would play because I was still getting the chance to play for Liverpool, but it just wasn't my position. I'd go through games wondering: 'What am I doing here?'

Inevitably, my form suffered as a result, and then the crowd started getting on my back. It was the beginning of the end for me.

The most high-profile mistake I made was in a League Cup game we played against Lou Macari's Stoke City at Anfield in September 1991. We ended up drawing 2-2 after conceding from a header at a corner in the first half and then, late on, directly from my error. I under-hit a back pass and Tony Kelly tucked it under Bruce to score. I'd been really struggling with my form anyway. It's on nights like that you wish no one had been on the Kop, and that the ground swallows you up and you can escape.

Ironically, it was one of the few games that my dad had actually attended and, afterwards, I was stood talking to him in the players' lounge when Graeme poked his head around the door, looked at me briefly, then disappeared.

I got in the following day, and straight away Graeme was on at me. "I thought you might have taken your mistake a bit more seriously," he said.

"What do you mean?"

"I saw you in the lounge having a drink."

"I wasn't. I was standing talking to my dad, waiting for the crowd to go so that I could go home."

Silence. But he wasn't finished.

"Anyway, I know you cost us the second goal, but I thought it was your fault for the first as well."

This wasn't going particularly well. I wasn't big on confrontation, but I was determined to stand up for myself. "I wasn't down to mark their man who scored," I replied, trying to stay as calm as I could.

In many respects, whether I'd continued arguing the point or not that morning was hardly the point. Fighting my corner wouldn't have amounted to anything. I knew my Liverpool dream was unravelling.

As a footballer, you know you are going to make mistakes in games. Most goals originate from someone's mistake but, like a golfer who suffers from the yips, one stray pass or poor piece of control can quickly snowball into something more serious. It becomes a vicious circle if you are not careful. You make a mistake, hear the groans of the crowd, maybe someone shouting "Fuck off, Ablett," and the next time you get the ball or face an opponent there is a sense of anxiety gripping you.

I know that says something about my ability, and mentality, as a player in a team that routinely hit the heights, but it is a horrendous feeling becoming a target for the boo boys. For one thing, you feel it a lot more being a local lad because you are representing so many people – people like you. And there is no escape half the time.

Being truthful, I couldn't handle what was going on. My game felt as if it was disintegrating around me. I'd been hauled out of my comfort zone and asked to play in positions where I wasn't at home, and things had gone from bad to worse. Increasingly, I was frightened to touch the ball; frightened to get involved in case I made another mistake.

My performances reflected as much. Form drained away completely, my displays becoming poorer and poorer and, as a result, the crowd got at me more and more. Up until that point in my career I'd always felt that Saturday afternoons were an opportunity to go out and show what I could do. Everything was geared towards kick-off and the chance to showcase everything I was good at. Not any more. Now, Saturdays had become less of an opportunity and more of an ordeal. My form stunk. Maybe if I'd been playing in a position where I was more comfortable things might have been different – maybe, or maybe not – but this was like asking John Barnes to start playing right-back. Actually, thinking about it, he was such a natural he might have done that supremely well.

But for someone who had been playing centre-back for years, to suddenly be asked to go and fill in on the left of midfield, trying to beat opposing full-backs on the outside and fling accurate crosses into the box...well, that was hard. There was no help offered up by the coaching staff or fellow players. No advice was offered. No one really said anything about the situation. Of course, my team-mates geed me up on match days, but I was letting them down and the last thing I wanted to be was the side's weakest link.

As for the abuse, it was merciless. It reached the stage where I would avoid walking down Church Street into Liverpool city centre, past all the market stalls, because I knew every step I took would be accompanied by a chorus of abuse.

It wasn't particularly nasty. But when you hear someone you've never met before telling you you're "shite" for the 20th time, you do start to wonder why you are putting yourself through it. 'I don't need this,' I thought, so I stayed out of the way waiting for things to settle down. The problem was they never really did.

The more groans and boos I heard, the more I went into my shell. I was lost, alone.

As it was, things were changing at Liverpool anyway. The balance of the team was shifting. Graeme had brought in Nicky Tanner and Mike Marsh was coming through while, at the same time, he was actively looking to move on one or two of the older players he had inherited. The upheaval was all too much, too soon in my opinion. Over a longer period of time, his approach could have possibly been more successful. But Liverpool did not need the sort of revolution he was trying to implement at the club.

In fairness to Graeme, I did sign a new four-year deal in the November of 1991 when he was manager but, even as I was putting pen to paper, I was thinking to myself that it would be a miracle if I saw that out. One Friday morning in early January, he pulled me to one side in the old pavilion at Melwood. He said he had received an offer from a club for me, and asked if I would be interested in going.

"It depends who it is," I said.

"I'm not telling you who it is unless you say you want to go," was Graeme's response.

"So what are you telling me?"

"Well you are falling down the pecking order here, you are behind Nicky Tanner..."

That served as a thunderclap. As much as I got on with Nick – we had played in the reserves together – I just couldn't understand how he was in the team at centre-half ahead of me. Surely I was worth more.

Graeme continued: "You will be third or fourth choice here, you'll make some of my squads and not others. It's up to you. What do you want to do?"

As he said those words I knew that was it. My Liverpool career was over. I could have tried to ride it out, safe in the knowledge that I had my long-term contract to fall back upon, but he was the manager and if I was not part of his plans, then what was the point in staying? I thought I might as well go and play for someone who was going to appreciate me. That's the reality of football. And that was my reality. There was no choice to be made, though I needed to know who had expressed an interest in me first. Someone out there clearly still had faith in my ability.

"If you are telling me I have no real option, then I'll listen to who it is," I said.

"It's Howard Kendall. Everton want you."

And so the lad who had grown up as a Liverpool fan but was now getting battered every other week by his fellow supporters, whether I was sinking on the pitch or strolling through my hometown, decided to do the 'simple' thing and move across the city to the club's biggest rivals. Whatever decisions I have made in my life, no one can ever accuse me of taking the easy option. This was out of the frying pan and into the fire.

9

—

Feeling Blue

Howard had always liked me. When he was Manchester City manager, he'd once bumped into me and said if I ever wanted a move, no matter where he was, he would take me. There was no great friendship between us, no obvious link, but I just found he was someone who was very personable. He was someone I liked and could get along with.

In that sense he was completely different to Graeme. The appeal of playing for someone who actually wanted me was too hard to resist. Plus, this was the chance to revert back to a position that I was comfortable playing in. There was a brief chat on the phone and Howard said that, for him, I would play left-back or centre-half. That was reassuring to hear, to be honest. I went to have a medical one Friday night in Rodney Street with the club physio, Les Helm, and there were no problems. I then met Howard in the Moat House Hotel in Liverpool city centre to discuss a few other things.

I had just signed a contract for Liverpool not long previously, so

Everton just kept me on the same money. The deal was £2,000-a-week, the most I had ever earned as a player up to that time. There was a pretty big discrepancy between that and what people like John Barnes and Peter Beardsley were earning, which was probably in the region of £4,000 to £5,000-a-week. But they were the stars, brought in for what were eye-watering fees back then. I was just the local kid who had come up through the ranks and was happy to pull on a shirt. Still, considering I had played in the 1988 FA Cup final while earning £600-a-week, it wasn't too bad at all.

Soon there would be a nice little bonus as well. Despite having a medical the night before, I was in the Liverpool squad for a game against Luton Town at Anfield on 11 January but, not particularly surprisingly, I didn't make the cut for the line-up.

Everton were playing Manchester United on the same Saturday and Howard had suggested we meet at Bellefield, Everton's training ground in West Derby, at 7pm that night to finalise everything. I was keen to keep the move hush-hush at that stage and, although Bellefield was only a mile or so away from Melwood, I knew it wouldn't be particularly busy at that time so it seemed the perfect place to meet.

Everton lost 1-0 at Old Trafford and I knew it wouldn't take Howard long to arrive back on Merseyside and for the deal to be completed. I was waiting in my car outside the training ground, when I suddenly saw the team bus come round the corner and pull up next to me. 'Howard, what have you done to me?' I thought to myself. So much for keeping things quiet.

The players filed off the coach, peering into my car and seeing me sat there. I just nodded back sheepishly, embarrassed that my move across the city boundaries was being witnessed by all my prospective new team-mates. Howard just laughed it off. He took me up to his office, which was about the size of a broom cupboard, and he poured a little drink for us both.

"Listen. I've got to ring Graeme," he said, picking up the phone and punching in Graeme's number. "Graeme, it's Howard. I've spoken to Gary. He doesn't want to do the deal." He had a twinkle in his eye as he said that, moving the phone away from his mouth, covering the handset and smiling and winking at me across the desk while I just looked on, astonished. What the hell was he up to? I'd just told him I'd sign, no problem.

"What do you mean he doesn't want to do the deal?" I could hear Graeme barking back down the line.

"You're not offering him enough to go."

"How much does he want?"

"Another £25,000."

Howard moved the phone away from his mouth again. This time I was smiling.

There was a pause. "Okay, he can have it," said Graeme.

Just like that, Howard had got me an extra £25,000. Unbelievable. Although, in one respect, it showed how desperate Graeme was to get rid of me. Howard had never discussed anything with me about what he did. He just did it off his own bat, and I certainly wasn't complaining. Goodness knows how many clubs he tried it on with like that. But he wasn't finished yet.

"Right lad, what are you doing now?" added Howard. "Do you fancy going into Southport then for a night out?"

"I live in the south end, Howard. I'd better get home to be fair." The money his opportunism had earned me went straight into my pension but, as soon as he did that for me, I thought he was the type of manager I wanted to play for. I would give him everything. Nothing has changed from that day to this. I love the bones of the man and hear from him every so often. He always has a kind word, always telling me I'll beat this terrible disease. I will always like being in his company.

Yet, despite all the warmth Howard showed me from the start, this wasn't an easy move to make. Peter Beardsley had been sold by Graeme a few months earlier and turned up at Everton, but he didn't bring the baggage of being a local boy with him. There was a respect for Peter as well. Liverpool fans didn't particularly want him to go, and Evertonians knew they were getting a player who had enjoyed a brilliant career.

In contrast, Liverpool supporters couldn't wait to see the back of me after my form had unravelled, and Everton fans were unimpressed at the prospect of signing what was, I suppose, a reject from their bitter rivals. I knew there would be abuse. I'm not soft. But I genuinely didn't anticipate the level of vitriol that was aimed at me.

You could be walking down the street, a car would go past and someone would shout: "Fuck off, Ablett." Or I'd get called a "shitbag", which was actually one of the tamer insults flung my way. It got to the stage where I couldn't tell who was abusing me: Evertonians or Liverpudlians. It felt like a free-for-all. I have to say my family escaped being targeted themselves. Certainly, my dad or brother has never mentioned falling victim to the kind of abuse I was getting. I suppose football has changed since then, though. Players' families are caught up in all the hoopla that goes with the game these days, people are famous for whom they are married to and everyone is a celebrity.

The media didn't help, either, with the local radio stations, rather than the press, stirring things up as though I had committed some sort of heinous crime. To be honest, I thought people would get over it, but it took time – far longer than I had imagined. I wasn't going to give in, though. The move afforded me the chance to play and gain some respect. I knew I had to get the Everton players on side, the Everton fans on side and I knew I had to prove something to Graeme. I had to show him that he'd been wrong to let me go.

* * * * * * * * * * * * * * * *

My debut for Everton came in a league game at Goodison Park against Nottingham Forest about a week after I had joined. I was nervous, but it was a different type of nerves to those I had ever experienced at Liverpool. I didn't doubt my own ability this time round, but I was just anxious to get off to a good start. I was desperate to get a solid performance behind me and show the fans that, just maybe, Howard hadn't signed a bum after all.

While we were getting changed I pulled Neville Southall in the dressing room and asked him to try and give me an early touch of the ball if he could. "I just want to get settled," I said. "Roll the ball out to me if you can."

So out we went on to the pitch at Goodison Park, me searching for that reassuring first involvement and big Neville apparently playing ball. Forest launched an early attack and a cross came over, which he duly plucked out of the air with consummate ease. This was my chance. I peeled off straight away and made a run wide into the left-back position, making myself available for Neville to find me and start a counter-attack. What followed was a lesson in being careful about just what you wish for...

He tried to find me alright but, when he launched the ball at me, it was like one of Shane Warne's googlies – one pitched into a foot hole just in front of the popping crease. The ball helpfully bounced about a yard in front of me. You can guess the rest: I put my leg out to trap it, the ball reared up and hit my knee, rebounding straight into the Bullens Road stand. Goodison Park let out a collective groan as if all those present were asking themselves: 'Jesus Christ, what have we fuckin' gone and got here, then?'

As I jogged back into position, ready to defend the throw-in I glanced back towards Neville. He was stood in his penalty area with just a hint of a smile twitching across his face. At half-time I pulled him again. "Thanks for that," I said. He just laughed. That was just Neville.

Something else I had to learn about. I'd played with Bruce Grobbelaar at Liverpool, an eccentric in his own way, but even he wouldn't have done that to the new boy in the team. But Neville was just a character to grow accustomed to.

I actually found things far more relaxed and comfortable at Everton. I may have played the best football of my career at Liverpool because, across Stanley Park, I'd been playing with better players. But, being truthful, I enjoyed my time at Everton far more. There wasn't the same pressure. The spotlight wasn't as intense on the club, and that suited me down to the ground.

I am not stupid – I know what that says about me as a player. I was happier because I suppose I had found my level away from the super-stars. For the Liverpool supporters who turned on me, maybe this was proof that, in the long run, I wasn't right for them. But I had never claimed to be one of Liverpool's best-ever players. If you go into the club's new offices in Chapel Street in the city centre, there is a roll of honour on the wall and my name is first. But I'm more than aware that it's been listed in alphabetical order rather than order of importance. I can accept that.

If you lost a game with Liverpool, the fall-out was huge. There'd be an inquest in the media and from the coaches. Imagine the intensity of it all if you then went on to fail to win a few games on the spin. You were expected to win cups and fill the trophy cabinet ever year. Season after season after season.

At Everton, a big club in its own right, there just wasn't that same pressure. After their purple patch in the mid-1980s, they were on the way down and even a mid-table finish wasn't perceived as being disas-trous. If you managed a decent cup run, then the season was actually considered to have been something of a success.

Don't get me wrong: all the players there wanted to win. When you have Neville in your dressing room, together with the likes of Dave

Watson, there was no cutting corners. Yet there simply wasn't the same level of expectation. I felt more comfortable within the group as well, so I would go out a lot more. And we used to have a laugh.

I remember one Christmas later in my time there we had a fancy dress party at the Continental. I think I'd gone as a German Gestapo officer or something similarly clichéd. Mark Ward was there, and one of his mates had what was supposed to be a cap gun with him. Technically it was a toy gun, but when Wardy aimed it at Barry Horne and fired, Barry ended up flying half-way across the club. It was just Wardy messing about, and everyone burst out laughing until one or two of us said: "Jesus, what's gone on here?"

Barry had come dressed as a priest, so you can imagine the scene: he's lying on his back, seven sheets to the wind, with a hole smouldering in his chest. We threw ale over him to get rid of the smoke, dusted him down and then carried on drinking.

Barry seemed too shocked to have a real go, and I think Wardy was taken aback by how powerful this toy gun was. He certainly didn't take aim again that night, that's for sure.

The Everton players were just a good, tightly-knit group. You didn't have to be on your guard with them – cap guns aside, clearly – or wary of doing the wrong thing and being battered mercilessly for it. I could finally be myself.

The medals I won at Liverpool mean everything to me. That is what you come into the game for. You can keep your fancy cars and £50,000-a-week wage packages which, these days, run-of-the-mill players who never get a sniff of silverware can expect to enjoy. The fanciest car I ever had as a player was an Escort convertible or a Mercedes. That side of things didn't interest me. But at Everton, I found something else: a sense of belonging.

Having Howard at the helm helped. You could have a laugh with Kenny Dalglish, while Graeme wanted to fight all the time. But Howard was relaxed, and so the club was relaxed, too, but not in a bad way. He was still sharp, but he enjoyed himself.

On away trips he would sit at the front of the coach, going over his plans for the game in his head. On the way home, win, lose or draw, he would be at the back: trousers off, sitting in his silk boxer shorts and shirt playing cards with the lads. We played a game called Aces to Kings and there was Howard, me, John Ebbrell, Ian Snodin, the kit man Jimmy Martin and one or two others. Howard would have a bottle of champagne between his feet and, if he ran out, he'd shout someone to get another bottle from the front.

They played for pennies rather than pounds. It was just a way of unwinding after a game, and nothing that would upset the harmony of the squad whereby someone would end up hundreds of pounds out of pocket by the time the coach arrived back home.

It was just his way of relaxing. I know from my own spell in charge of Stockport County the stress you feel when you are a manager, and Howard used to wind down with a game of cards and a drink.

I remember us coming back from a London game one Saturday and we had drunk the bus dry by Birmingham. Howard had been sent over some crates of red wine from friends in Bilbao, people he'd got to know when he had managed there, and the bottles were meant to be a present for his wife. He'd stored them in the lock-ups on the side of the coach and, realising there was no more booze on board, he ordered the coach to pull over on the hard shoulder. Someone went to fetch the red wine and we carried on drinking. I'm not sure how his wife took it. Actually, this is probably the first she'd know about it.

We went on a pre-season trip to Switzerland one year and I'd been given the short straw of rooming with Maurice Johnston. I liked Maurice a lot, but he always wanted to be doing something and didn't like just sitting around. We'd been ordered to stay in our rooms after lunch and rest because we were playing a match against a local side that night but, predictably, he couldn't settle.

We could only have been back half-an-hour when he decided he was hungry. "I need some chocolate or crisps," he said to me, before sticking his head out the door and shouting down the corridor.

"Hey," he bellowed.

Howard answered. "What's going on?"

"Boss, I'm starving. I need something to eat."

Howard asked who he was rooming with and so Maurice shouted back: "Gary Ablett."

"Right, you two come with me."

Next minute, Howard is marching us down the main street in this Swiss town to a little bar. We spent two-and-a-half hours having a drink and eating ham sandwiches that Howard would conjure from his pocket. "You two aren't playing tonight," he told us. That was just the way he was.

If it sounds like there was a lot of alcohol involved in those days, it was simply because that was still part of the culture. You wouldn't get away with it these days, of course.

Howard still cared deeply about winning. One of my first-ever trips with the club was to Bilbao during an international break. We were flying on to Magaluf for a bit of team bonding, but first we had the match to play. The locals made a fuss of Howard from his stint in the city and he wanted to show he was still a good manager.

But the first half was dismal. We came in at 0-0 having barely managed an attack of note and, when we were in the changing rooms, he made it known to us all that he wasn't happy. "Come on, time to get your fucking fingers out and do a little," he yelled at us, before sending us back out for the second half.

Stuart Barlow and Tony Cottee scored in the second half and we won 2-0. Howard was made up. After the final whistle, there was a bottle of champagne by everyone's peg in the changing room and he told the club secretary, Jim Greenwood, to sort the lads out. Jim gave us £250 cash each for when we went to Magaluf. That was the type of manager Howard was. If you looked after him, he would look after you. Players will give a bit more for a manager they think is on their side and Howard knew that. He worked on that. At times he would rant and rave, but not very often. On occasions, he would 'create' a row just to send a message to the dressing room.

There was one time when we went to Crystal Palace and he pulled me and Dave Watson to one side. "You've been magnificent for me this past month, but I'm going to tear into you in front of the other players," he said. "I need a reaction from them and the best way is by bollocking you two."

We just went along with it. Kick-off loomed and Howard started off with his speech, ripping into us. "Listen," he said, pointing at Waggy and me. "You've got to do better and start doing more for your team-mates. Lift your fucking standards." We duly won 2-0 with goals from Matt Jackson and Peter Beardsley, so I suppose the psychology worked.

I loved my time under him, and he could still play. He'd give you a run for your money in a game of head tennis or whatever. Every morning, Howard would be in the gym playing one or two touch with Colin Harvey on his team.

There is a whole generation of Everton supporters who probably don't fully appreciate Howard and what he did for the club. Yet, when you consider that he pushed Liverpool in the 1980s and, for a brief spell, broke their dominance, it speaks volumes about what a fine manager he was. Everton played such attractive football then as well: Kevin Ratcliffe at the back, Peter Reid and Paul Bracewell in central midfield, Trevor Steven on the right and Sharpy in attack. They were a great team and, but for the European ban on clubs in the aftermath of the Heysel disaster, could well have ruled Europe.

Howard pokes fun at himself, telling the story about how he "went away to get 'dried out' and came back with Rideout", but it is written large in history that he's Everton's most successful-ever manager, and I don't think his record will be beaten any time soon, even with all the fine work David Moyes has done over the last decade.

It obviously frustrated him that the league championships, FA Cup and the European Cup-Winners' Cup he had won first time around couldn't be repeated during his second spell in charge and that, invariably, we had memorable wins rather than memorable seasons. But the balance of power had tipped since the 1980s.

Even so, we went to Old Trafford at the start of the 1992/93 season and won 3-0. Peter Beardsley, Robert Warzycha and Maurice scored. The Stretford End was getting done up at the time, and we got absolutely battered – we had tin hats on at the back. Howard picked quite an attack-minded team and fortune favoured him that day.

Another game that sticks in my mind was my first Merseyside derby as an Everton player at Goodison in December 1992. There was plenty riding on that game for me: earning the respect of both sets of fans for starters, as well as the Liverpool staff, especially Graeme. That was a huge motivation for me to show him that, if I was played in my proper position, I could do well.

Mark Wright opened the scoring in the second half for Liverpool, but within a minute Maurice had scored to equalise. Then, with time running out, Peter scored the winner and we won 2-1. The din was tremendous. Goodison Park erupted and there a real sense of triumphalism inside the ground. Afterwards there was a just a massive sense of relief for me. I'd played my part in the goal by stepping off the line and picking out Peter with a pass before he took a touch and smashed the ball into the bottom corner.

If it was a big moment for him, then I felt 10ft tall. 'Take that', I thought. I knew I wasn't a dud, and maybe one or two others would have the same opinion. It was just a shame there weren't a few more days like that.

Howard left a year after I had arrived after clashing with the board in December 1993. They refused to back him over the signing of Dion Dublin from Manchester United so he walked away from the job. It was bitterly disappointing for me because he was the reason I had gone to Everton in the first place and he was the manager I had wanted to play for. Football's football though. It happens, and you have to get on with it. Someone else comes in and, if you spend all your time hankering after his predecessor then, pretty soon, you'll be out the door, too.

I had other things going on in my life, anyway. My first marriage had broken up and it was around the time that Howard left that I met Jacqueline. Her mum and dad used to own a caravan at a place called The Riverside in Tarleton about half-an-hour from Liverpool, not far from Preston. It was a place where we could come away after matches and just relax. No one knew me up there, no one would bother me. I could come away and have a drink.

Jacqueline came from a big family and at weekends, we'd all meet up. One Sunday morning at about 10am, everyone was still waking up when there was a knock on the caravan door. I shouted: "Who's that?"

A fella said he was so and so from the News of the World and that he wanted to come in for a chat. "What do you want to talk about?" I said, racking my brains over what it could be.

"We believe you are living in a caravan with your girlfriend and just want to talk to you about it."

"Piss off. Don't be so soft. Leave us alone."

The fella pushed a card under the door before he left, obviously thinking I would be back in touch. I phoned my agent and solicitor after the journalist had disappeared and they told me to ask for £50,000 to sell my story. Not surprisingly, when I did, I didn't hear back.

What was the story, anyway? They hadn't done their homework correctly. Firstly, I wasn't living in the caravan and, secondly, I was single so it was hardly the love rat story they presumably wanted. I didn't want to be splashed across the papers and, after a few weeks had elapsed, I thought nothing more of my brush with the tabloids.

* * * * * * * * * * * * * * * * *

Mike Walker's time in charge at Everton will hardly be remembered with any great fondness. Indeed, arguably the best result he ever achieved at Goodison Park was a 5-1 win there in September 1993 when he was still in charge of Norwich City, and Efan Ekoku scored four times. It was a win that no doubt helped him to get the job as Howard's successor, but he never came close to repeating that high.

You could argue he was trying to broaden our minds as players with the methods he tried to introduce, but we just never took to him. He wanted us to play like Norwich, whom he had helped challenge for the league title in the first year of the Premier League – they eventually finished third – and then led to a famous UEFA Cup elimination of Bayern Munich, knocking the ball around all nicely-nicely.

There were code names and nicknames – such as 'Sid' or 'Jack' – for certain things he wanted us to do on the pitch, like step-overs, and all this was alien to our dressing room. If he had been an arsehole the fact that his methods weren't working would have been easier to take, but actually he was a nice fella, by and large.

He was a bit of a sun worshipper who would have the sleeves on his t-shirt rolled up and his shorts rolled up whenever it wasn't raining. He also liked a drink with the lads, but I just think he wasn't the right fit for Everton. It happens – just look at Roy Hodgson. He's had a successful career in coaching for 30-plus years, but he was a square peg in a round hole at Liverpool and didn't really understand what the job was all about. It was a similar story for Mike, and it just never quite felt right under him.

There was never any question of the lads not trying. It was more simply a case of: 'What's he going on about?'

On the pitch, everything was a struggle. From around Christmas time in the 1993/94 season, we realised that we were in a battle for survival. This was a new experience for everyone, especially me. When you are fighting to win a league title there is pressure, but it is different to the suffocating sense you feel when you are trying to keep your head above water at the other end of the table.

Chasing silverware fills you with positive emotions, you're generally on a roll, winning matches, getting praise and looking to create landmarks that will stand the test of time. At Everton we were looking to avoid a piece of unwanted history. No one wanted to be labelled with the tag of having been part of the team that took Everton out of the top flight for the first time since 1951, and we all knew we had a responsibility to ensure that didn't happen. But, at the same time, you can find yourself powerless to prevent yourself being dragged deeper and deeper into the mire.

We had a decent team, but it was just not working under Mike. We arrived at that final game of the season against Wimbledon knowing another defeat would more than likely relegate us. Even then, we needed other results to go our way, with Oldham Athletic facing Norwich City and Sheffield United at Chelsea.

It was a surreal day from start to finish. Wimbledon's team coach had been set on fire and burnt out at their team hotel on Merseyside the night before the game, but if that was done by Evertonians to try and intimidate them then they had probably picked the wrong opposition. The Park End stand was being constructed then, so Goodison was only full on three sides for arguably one of the biggest games in the club's history and it made for a slightly surreal atmosphere. Not that everyone was bothered about whether Everton stayed up or not.

While some supporters had climbed trees in Stanley Park and were peering across a busy road and through the gaps in a stand that was half-built to catch a glimpse of the game, I remember Dave Watson saying he'd seen a bus go past with a fella on the top deck just reading his paper. He was oblivious to the fact Everton's future rested on 90 minutes against the original Crazy Gang.

I don't remember Mike giving any big speeches before kick-off. We knew what we had to do, we didn't particularly need any glib sound-bites. When you faced Wimbledon, you knew you had to match them in terms of the spirit they had in bucket loads, first of all. There were no secrets. If you did that, you might have a chance.

But we got off to a particularly poor start that Saturday afternoon, presumably due to the tension and what was at stake. Dean Hold-sworth scored early on with a penalty and then another shot hit me and bobbled into the corner for an own goal. Being truthful, I thought that was it. I thought I'd unwittingly had a hand in the goal that would send Everton tumbling out of the top flight. At 2-0 down, I just didn't see how we could possibly get back into the game.

You might have expected Goodison to be like a morgue at that point, but the atmosphere was actually still spine-tingling and we grabbed a lifeline just before half-time with a goal from the penalty spot from Graham Stuart. That gave us hope, something to cling to, and some momentum going into the second period. Even so, there was still a sense of disbelief when Barry Horne smashed one in from 25 yards to make it 2-2. Players like Barry and John Ebbrell were real heroes that day. They really spurred the rest of us on, digging deep and being as aggressive as they could, making sure that if Vinnie Jones put his foot in for a tackle, they'd be there, too.

If I am honest, I am still not sure about the third goal. It would be wrong for me to say that I thought Hans Segers had deliberately let it in at the time. No one thought that. No one thought there was any-thing out of the ordinary about how Graham Stuart's shot had slipped under his body and into the back of the net. At the time, all you could think about was the noise and the emotion that we may just have saved ourselves from the drop.

However, with the subsequent publicity that game has received and the allegations of match fixing, you do wonder. In the first half, I had taken a free-kick and put everything into the shot, catching it just right. Hans plucked it out of the air as if he was picking cherries. Fast forward to Graham's shot later on and, well, all I will say is perhaps he could have done better...

Wimbledon had an air about them that day. I liked Vinnie Jones. He was just a down to earth lad in my view, and I remember seeing him in the players' lounge afterwards. He and some of the other Wimbledon lads were smoking these huge cigars and drinking pints. I thought it was strange, as they'd just got beat. Then again, it was the final game of the season and what a season they had enjoyed. They had finished sixth and, once again, proved that they were more than simply a bunch of cloggers.

For us, there was cause to let off steam rather than celebrate. Having spent most of the afternoon staring at disaster, the final whistle simply brought an overwhelming feeling of relief. Utter relief. We wouldn't be saddled with the tag of having taken Everton down. Even a draw wouldn't have been good enough that day, but it was Sheffield United who went down instead after they conceded a last-minute goal to lose at Chelsea. Oldham also perished after only drawing at Norwich. We had survived.

But there was no huge celebration, no club party or anything. What was there to really celebrate, anyway? A club like Everton shouldn't have been in that position, scrapping for its life, although sadly it wasn't the only time Evertonians saw a last-day escape. How we managed to get out of the hole we were in, I'm still not totally sure. Certain individuals will take that to the grave with themselves.

I just wanted to get away and forget about everything that summer, to just chill out. It was my first holiday with Jacqueline and we went to Cyprus, though my old friends at the 'News of the World' ensured it wasn't quite the relaxing time I'd imagined. While I was away, I got a message that the article about myself, Jacqueline and the caravan would be going in the paper. 'Oh shit,' I thought. I'd not done anything wrong, but I just didn't need the hassle.

Sunday came and I was lying on a lounger reading the paper when I came to this double-page article. I peered over the top of the paper to see where Jacqueline was. "Have you seen this?" I asked her, knowing full well she hadn't. As it turned out, Jacqueline's mum was more upset that the article said her caravan had no toilet or hot water than about her daughter getting involved with me.

We'd made friends with quite a lot of people out in Cyprus. Lloyd McGrath, who used to play for Coventry, and Mike Sheron, the ex-Manchester City striker, were there, and the people who ran the bar we went to were massive Liverpool fans.

That Sunday night we went out and the bar owners had baked a cake for us. On it was a map of Cyprus and there, in the middle of the map, was a cut-out of a caravan.

10

Got Any Garys?

To different people I have come to mean different things. Some see me just as a footballer who enjoyed a career on either side of the Liverpool city divide. To others I am considered a husband, a father and now, I suppose, a cancer sufferer. But, for a spell, it seemed as if I was in danger of becoming better known for drugs more than anything else. Not that I have ever touched them.

The fact that my father and brother were both with the police force meant they were involved in surveillance operations in the late 1980s and early 1990s, and it was them who first picked up on the reality that dealers were constantly referring to me in the conversations that were being monitored. Whether they were talking to their suppliers or their buyers, my name would pop up. I guess their first reaction might have been to wonder if their Gary had a secret other life overseeing the criminal underworld on Merseyside. Thankfully, they soon realised that I was being used – used as rhyming slang for ecstasy tablets. "Got any Gary Abletts – tablets?"

My dad phoned me one day and said people were going into clubs in Liverpool on Friday and Saturday nights asking if anyone "had any Garys". Back when I had been setting out on my career as a footballer, the prospect of half the youngsters in the city having my name on the tip of their tongue would no doubt have appealed to me. Not in these circumstances, though.

Sometimes even now I'll go on Twitter – Scarlet is responsible for bringing me up to speed with social networking sites because she was fed up with messages asking 'how I am' coming through to her account – and there are people still banging on about it. Idiots.

I'd prefer to hope that, in time, I might be better remembered for creating a slice of history in Merseyside football. My moment came at the giddy finale to the 1994/95 season. That campaign had ended in stark contrast to how it had begun. I hadn't been surprised that Mike Walker had been given the chance to go into the new season as manager. Yes, everyone in the dressing room felt things just weren't right under him, but maybe the Everton board were blinded to that by the sheer drama and relief of our great escape against Wimbledon on the previous season's last afternoon.

The reality was, of course, that our miraculous survival at Sheffield United's expense had not been down to Mike at all. It had been born of the players' drive, determination and character and, as it later transpired, perhaps an unexpected helping hand from Hans Segers. If the board had recognised that, they might have acted. As it was they didn't but, pretty soon, it was clear they would have no choice but to do something about it.

A home draw on the opening day against Aston Villa may have hinted that better times lay ahead, but it was a false dawn. We lost at Tottenham Hotspur, were battered 4-0 by Manchester City, lost to Nottingham Forest at Goodison Park and then were turned over comfortably by Blackburn Rovers. After 14 games of the season, we were rooted to the foot of the Premier League table. Our record in all competitions going into the home match with West Ham United was embarrassing reading: P14, W0, D5, L9, GF 11, GA 28. We had just four points to show for our endeavours in the league. It was pathetic stuff.

I had missed some of that dismal run but, watching from the side-lines, I thought we should have won some of those matches. We had good players in our squad and the first team looked strong and solid. But, for whatever reason, we weren't clicking and when that happens, the manager invariably carries the can.

West Ham arrived at Goodison Park on 1 November and you could sense the anxiety around the ground. Our strikers hadn't really been firing and Tony Cottee was lining up against us, having moved back to Upton Park in a swap deal involving David Burrows after just three games of the season. The manager had obviously brought in Bugsy, another former Liverpool team-mate of mine, to put pressure on me. David Unsworth was also emerging through the ranks and forcing his way into the team, too, and it seemed like I was seen as the weak link in the boss's mind.

Mike should have had more faith. After all, I had scored in his first league game in charge – a 6-2 win over Swindon – pouncing on a loose ball in front of the Gwladys Street and slamming my shot into the net. I was deadly from six yards, and so it proved again that evening against the Hammers. A diving header brought us our first win of the campaign in front of 28,338 fans on a Tuesday night. The fact that the opening-day gate against Villa, albeit for a Saturday fixture, had been over 35,000 just showed how demoralising following Everton at the start of that season had become. It had been unremitting misery for the supporters, many of whom had clearly decided they could not take any more.

The win over West Ham might have suggested we were about to

kick-start our campaign but, rather than proving a turning point in our season, we quickly slipped back into poor habits. We went to Norwich, of all places, a few days later – they would go on to be relegated that season – and played out a dire 0-0 draw. Shortly afterwards the Everton chairman, Peter Johnson, sacked Mike, suggesting he had been the common denominator for both sides' failings that afternoon. I guess he had a point.

There was no mourning the end of his tenure inside the dressing room. It is one thing getting a sleepy club like Norwich punching above their weight, but Everton was a step up and a different type of pressure again. The need for a fresh start had become pretty obvious by then, and there was a realisation that, this time around, we wouldn't even get to the final game of the season with something still to play for. The way we were going, following the worst start in the club's history, we would most likely have been relegated by March.

* * * * * * * * * * * * * * * *

I still see and speak to Joe Royle quite a bit. He has visited my house numerous times during the illness, always geeing me up and reminding me to keep fighting. He has this great knack of being able to put a smile on my face, even when I feel like a bag of shite. In that sense, nothing has changed from the day he walked into Everton as Mike Walker's replacement. Now we had a proper manager in charge. The effect was like flicking a switch.

It tells you a lot about Joe's personality and qualities that the first thing he did when he came in was speak to the senior players about what had been going on, and what we needed to put right. Individually, we were called to see him, myself included. "We just need to get back to basics," I told him. "Being hard to beat. The players are better than we have been showing."

I think that was the general consensus from all of the lads in the dressing room. Neville, Dave Watson, Joe Parkinson and Barry Horne will all have said pretty much the same as me. Joe listened and then made his own decisions, but by taking the time to talk to us he immediately invoked a sense of togetherness that had been missing.

His number two was Willie Donachie, who was into meditation and would always impress on you the need to think positively. He was a little dour, but a nice man at the same time. If Willie had been at Liverpool when I was struggling to believe in myself, wracked by nerves and the feeling I just didn't belong in this company, I think I would have struck up a good rapport with him. That's what I needed at that time in my career, someone who would tell me I was better than I gave myself credit for.

By the time I was at Everton, though, I was far more comfortable in my own skin, more mature and experienced. Someone who would stand up and take the lead when the situation demanded it, rather than someone who retreated into the background. If I had to put my finger on one of the secrets of Joe's success at Everton, it would be that he made us all feel like that.

His first game in charge was the Merseyside derby at Goodison Park, and Liverpool were the perfect opposition for us to make a statement about how we wanted the rest of the season to pan out. I suppose the one thing you can credit Mike Walker with was starting Duncan Ferguson's love affair with Everton. He had signed both him and Iain Durrant on loan from Glasgow Rangers in September 1994 just before he was sacked, and Duncan had quickly set about winning over the fans. To be fair, scoring the opening goal against Liverpool isn't a bad way to open your account for Everton, although his far post header told only half the story.

The previous day he had been arrested for drink driving in the city and locked up, but that was just Duncan. The perception that he was nuts is totally wrong. He'd been involved in a few scrapes, but because he didn't speak to the press they built him up into something he was not. He wasn't an ogre. He was actually just a nice, down to earth lad, but someone who could handle himself alright.

He was a much better player than people gave him credit for as well. Once, when I was doing one of my UEFA coaching licences, I spent some time with Steve Bould and Tony Adams and we got to talking about Duncan. They said there was a picture up when Highbury was still Arsenal's ground of Duncan jumping for a cross and, in the photograph, he's about two feet above the crossbar. He met the header full on and it was going nowhere but the corner of the net. It was an unbelievable photo. The fella had clearly made an impression on those guys, which said a lot about his talent and his ability to hold his own. An in-form Duncan Ferguson could strike fear into central defenders up and down the country.

We felt we could get at Liverpool. Apart from maybe Neil Ruddock and Mark Wright, they didn't really have anyone who would like to try and mix it up. To be blunt, we thought we could bully them. Duncan's opener set the tone, and Paul Rideout scored the second goal after a mistake by David James to cap what was a dream start for Joe. He had a win in his first game, a victory over bitter local rivals to rekindle the whole club's enthusiasm, and Everton had moved off the bottom of the table as well to the heady heights of 20th place. It was a start, and we never really looked back from that moment.

The tag 'The Dogs of War' was borne out of those early performances, and was a tribute to the likes of Parky, John Ebbrell and Barry Horne. If someone needed to put their foot in during a game, to wrest back the initiative or impose ourselves on a contest, those three would be fighting each other to be the first one there.

But they had more strings to their bow than simply kicking opponents. I firmly believe that other clubs misunderstood that and were ultimately fooled by 'The Dogs of War' theme. They thought Everton couldn't play football, and soon found out that we could. We lost only six more matches that season after Joe's arrival, and that wasn't just down to kicking teams off the park. Give Anders Limpar room and he would make you pay. Andy Hinchcliffe's supply line from the left wing to Duncan made them a potent partnership, and there were plenty of others who chipped in: Graham Stuart, Rideout, Daniel Amokachi.

Unfortunately, I was injured not long after Joe had taken over. We played Leeds at Goodison and won 3-0, but I didn't see out the game. Brian Deane came crashing down on me after one aerial challenge and crushed all the vertebrae and cartilage in my neck. I was stretchered off in agony after about 15-20 minutes and transferred by ambulance to a hospital by Sefton Park. X-rays revealed the cartilage had also come away from my rib cage and it was absolute torture to take deep breaths. As for moving to get comfy in bed, forget about it. I was in hospital for a week, and sidelined for much longer.

It was as if, overnight, I became injury prone around then. As I completed my recovery from the damage sustained against Leeds I slipped getting out of the bath in my apartment at Waterloo Dock. I caught my little toe on the skirting board in the bathroom, pushing it out at a hideous right angle, and ended up shouting the block down in excruciating pain. I actually played the following week after that incident. We put a foam cushion inside the boot to offer some comfort, and six painkilling jabs did the rest.

It was only when we did further tests, however, that it became apparent that a cancerous growth had eaten all the bone away and there was only cartilage left in my toe.

Everton booked me into a private hospital on the Wirral called Murrayfield and I ended up having a foot graft, with a cow bone used to make my toe stronger.

Of course, I've wondered since whether this was a warning sign of the situation I now find myself in, but as far as I am concerned they are not linked. I also had a cancerous growth removed from the side of my body, but on both occasions they were benign and I've been told they have nothing to do with the lymphoma I now have.

I certainly didn't think anything of it at the time. I was fit and healthy and the procedures didn't worry me. If the truth be told I thought nothing of it. I just wanted to get back playing for Everton.

When I came back from injury, Joe found a place for me in the team. We ended up ensuring we would stay up – against all the odds given how miserable our start to the season had been – with a win at Ipswich in our penultimate league game of the campaign. Paul Rideout scored the only goal to complete the dramatic transformation Joe had overseen. As impressive was the fact that, while he was in charge of the club, you felt Everton would never be scrambling around, fighting for their lives, ever again.

After the Ipswich game, I bumped into one of the lads who used to follow Everton everywhere – Les O'Hare. He asked if I wanted a lift back to Merseyside and I asked the gaffer if it was okay. I jumped in the car and noticed we were following signs for the local airfield. Instead of driving the 250 or so miles, we were flying back in his private plane – I was home in an hour. But I'd never do that again. Les didn't clamber behind the controls, but it wasn't the most pleasant of journeys and I was thinking that, if we managed to make it home in one piece, I'd make sure I'd be going back on the team coach in future. Of course, teams do it all the time now. If Liverpool play in London in midweek, they'll usually get the train down for the game and then fly home straight after the match.

I went straight home. There was no big celebration planned, even though staying up was something to be proud of considering where we had been at the start of November. Instead, to a man, everyone in that squad felt another achievement, one that would eclipse every-thing, was within our grasp.

From the very first rounds in the FA Cup that season, everyone had thought Everton would go out with a whimper. They thought we'd be so wrapped up in trying to remain in the Premier League that we wouldn't take the competition seriously. We'd field weakened teams, or take our eyes off the ball, and quickly revert just to scraping together a few more points to stay above the cut-off. The truth is that all those assumptions people made actually helped us. The confidence we took from progressing in the cup also helped us in the league.

I missed the win over Derby County in the third round and against Bristol City in the fourth, when Matt Jackson scored, but returned to the team for the next game against Norwich. It was after that match, as we were sat in the dressing room, that we sensed for the first time that momentum was building and building. We had thrashed them 5-0 and been brilliant, playing them off the park. Anders, Parky, Paul Rideout, Duncan and Graham Stuart all scored, and suddenly we felt like contenders.

On a terrible pitch at Goodison, Newcastle were dispatched in the quarter-final thanks to a goal from Waggy (Dave Watson). Now for the semi-final. Of course, that was where everything was meant to end. We were to face Tottenham Hotspur, and Manchester United were pitted against Crystal Palace in the other semi. The watching world apparently wanted the so-called 'Dream Final' to be United versus Spurs. Fergie's champions against Gerry Francis' free-flowing, Jurgen Klinsmann-inspired Londoners. That was the glamour tie.

Yet, if ever one game dispelled the myth that Everton were merely a limited if wholehearted team, it was the Spurs semi-final match at Elland Road. The 'Dogs of War' bared their teeth that day, and our bite was ferocious.

The Grand National at Aintree had taken place the day before our semi-final and Royal Athlete was the winner. Royle's athletes weren't too bad themselves. Spurs had good players. There was class in their attacking ranks, with Darren Anderton, Teddy Sheringham, Klinsmann and Nick Barmby an attractive front-line. But we were just much, much better on the day. Matt scored, Graham Stuart got another and then Daniel Amokachi, who decided to substitute Paul Rideout while he was getting treatment off the pitch himself without Joe's permission, added two more. One of his brace came when I broke down the left and delivered the cross for him to convert. Stick your 'Dream Final'.

Afterwards, we met all the wives and girlfriends and had a party in town at a restaurant in Mathew Street. The celebrations hadn't really got going when there was a knock at the door and Vinny Samways appeared, standing with Neil Ruddock and his missus.

"Any chance Razor can join us?" he asked me.

I was close to Vinny, but I really didn't know how this would go down. This was Everton's night. My first thought was why Razor would even want to be celebrating with us? We'd just reached the FA Cup final while Liverpool weren't exactly tearing it up. They'd won the League Cup under Roy Evans that season and I was genuinely pleased for Roy, who had always been good to me. But, overall, they were only just emerging from the tough times they'd endured under Graeme.

Besides, can you imagine if that had made the papers at the time: 'Reds star parties with Joe's Blue Heroes' or 'Razor sings with the Blues'. There would have been uproar on the Kop. In truth, it was unusual for Liverpool and Everton players to mix at that time, but Razor is a one-off. He just wanted to have a drink and party.

"Let me ask Waggy," I said to Vinny.

I really thought Waggy might just say, "Tell him to fuck off", but he is sharp as a tack and was already thinking one step ahead. "Yes, he can come in," he said. "But he has to sing for the lads."

Razor, of course, isn't shy. He was straight up, belting out some number and keeping us all entertained. In the haze of the celebrations I'm not sure what it was he sang, but I'm pretty sure it wasn't "Que sera, sera, whatever will be, will be, we're going to Wem-ber-ley..." That was Everton's song of the moment. Whatever Razor did contribute on the mic, he was heckled like mad.

It was a great night and as it wore on, the lads started imagining we were walking up the steps at Wembley to be presented with the FA Cup itself. We were lifting these great big pots above our heads and, because we were all pretty drunk, banging them back down on the table. Unsurprisingly, the bottoms of the pots would smash into pieces although the bill for the damage was probably still less than the bill for the ale everyone drank.

Vinny was a close friend of mine and I still speak to him a lot now. We both had kids of a similar age when we were together at Everton – his son, Jay, is a little older than Scarlet – and when they were babies we used to take them to Southport on a Sunday afternoon and rock them to sleep in their car seats, while we had something to eat and a few drinks to unwind.

Unfortunately, he didn't have as good a relationship with Joe. I just don't think Joe fancied him as a player – but that's football. I just used to wind him up about not being in the team. That might seem harsh, taking the Micky out of one of your mates, but that is just how the banter went back then. I didn't mean anything by it. Given that we had been christened the 'Dogs of War', I guess it was apt that the attitude was dog eat dog.

11

People's Club

No one gave us a chance. We didn't have a prayer. Manchester United had beaten Crystal Palace after a replay in their semi-final and would be our opponents at Wembley. Pretty much everyone thought it would be a walkover for them. But I knew from Wimbledon back in 1988 that the favourites don't always come out on top.

We stayed at Sopwell House in St Albans in the build-up to the big day. I roomed with Duncan, who was struggling with injury at the time. But we all knew that, if we could get him on the pitch and play the ball to him in the right place, he would upset United. Even if he could only do that from the bench. I've got to say the atmosphere among the team was pretty relaxed. We knew they would have chances in the game, even though the likes of Eric Cantona and Andy Cole were missing, but if we defended well we'd surely get a chance ourselves? We had only conceded one goal en route to Wembley, and that was a Jurgen Klinsmann penalty in the semi-final which shouldn't have been given.

Joe came into his own that day. In the dressing room just before kick-off, he gave a great speech that, when boiled down, basically said: "Don't come back here after the match with any regrets." And so we didn't. We brought the FA Cup back with us instead.

I should actually have scored in the first half. Andy Hinchcliffe played a corner to the near post and, as I tried to get my head on it, the ball hit my shoulder and skimmed across the top of the bar. If I had caught it right, it would have gone in. As it was, that moment didn't cost us. Paul Rideout's header allowed us to get our noses in front and we put our bodies on the line after that to keep United at bay.

It would be wrong to single any one player out because everyone did their bit that day. So here is what I think of them all, my thoughts on Everton's class of '95...

Neville Southall:

Even then, he was still the best goalkeeper in the world in my opinion. Peter Schmeichel was up there, but when you saw Neville work day-to-day, the effort and commitment he put in to keep him at a certain level, it was unbelievable. He didn't go to the Cup final party afterwards and explained on television that, if anyone spent as much time with all of us as he did, then people would understand why he just wanted to go home. That was Nev. No one took umbridge or questioned him because you knew he did it on the pitch for you. He was ruthless in the dressing room, very cut-throat in his comments, and you had to roll with him and give him some back. But at the same time, he would do anything for you as well.

Matt Jackson:

We called him 'Floppy' because his arms and legs were all over the place, as though he was a puppet whose strings had been cut. He was a young lad when he arrived from Luton, but was a good player who weighed in with his fair share of goals. The left-foot, half volley against

Bristol City in the fourth round was an example of that. Of course, it was Matt's surging run, half the length of the Wembley pitch, that was crucial in the winning goal. Not only that, but the composure and vision he showed after it to pick out Graham Stuart with such a clever pass. We still keep in touch. I can go three months without speaking to him and then we'll have a catch-up. But it always feels like we spoke only the day before, there's never any awkwardness in the conversations. He's become a good friend. He's a bright lad. The only downside to him was that, along with Neville and Andy Hinchcliffe, he used to make up what was known as 'compost corner' in the dressing room. There was just crap everywhere you looked. And the smell...well, that stays with me to this day.

Dave Watson:

He was the one who held us together, that team's glue. Waggy kept the game simple. He headed it, kicked it, tackled it and weighed in with some important goals. He was someone you looked up to as an inspiration and thought: 'Yes, I'd go to war with him. He'll have my back.' I was in a Liverpool team alongside Alan Hansen, but Waggy is up there as the best I have played with. I can't remember a game where we came off thinking Waggy had been 'off it' that day. He was a seven/eight/nine out of 10 every game player. He was tough as anything and, if anyone deserved to lift the Cup that day, it was him.

David Unsworth:

He played particularly well in the Cup final and kept Mark Hughes quiet, which was no mean feat. We called him 'Rhino' and the physical battle he had with Hughes that day showed the nickname fitted him. There weren't many kids coming through at Everton at that time, but when you saw him in training you always thought he had a big chance of making it. He wanted to learn and wanted to better himself. He also wanted to get into the team and that meant a direct challenge to me and the others, but it never affected our relationship. If you fell out with everyone in your career who played in the same position as yourself, you'd never stop fighting. So, instead, you have to try and let it drive you on.

Graham Stuart:

We used to call him 'Nookie Bear' because of his wonky eyes, and 'Diamond' as well. He loved the craic and, while he was a bit quiet at first after coming up from London where he'd made his name at Chelsea, he soon joined in all the banter. He became part of the card school at the back of the bus with Howard on away games, and the fact that he still lives up this way now shows the warmth he has towards this area. He was a good player, who would always give his all. He helped keep Everton up and he should really have scored the winning goal in the Cup final, but it was his shot that came down off the crossbar that allowed Paul Rideout to become the hero. Not that Diamond lets Paul ever forget that he owed it all to him...

Barry Horne:

In any team, you have to trust your team-mates if you are going to get anywhere. When there's a battle out on the pitch, will he take a pass off you or will he hide? Will he still make tackles or will he simply fade into the background? Barry was unspectacular, but he always did his job and had the admiration of the dressing room for that. He was a 'Steady Eddie'. If it was there to be tackled, he tackled it. If it needed a simple pass, he gave a simple pass. He didn't over-complicate football and that was the key to his – and our – success that day.

Joe Parkinson:

He was like a warrior, one of the integral members of the 'Dogs of War', but don't take anything away from him: he could play as well. In many respects, that's the mix you want. Someone who is tough as nails and won't shirk a 50-50 or even a 40-60 with Roy Keane or Vinnie Jones, but at the same time someone who can spot a pass. It is a shame he got the knee injury at a stage in his career when people were talking about him as a possible England international. As a team-mate, he was top class.

Andy Hinchcliffe:

If I am being honest, I don't think he fulfilled the potential he had. Don't get me wrong, he played for England, but I think he could have been even better than he was. In the same way that I thought I needed help at Liverpool, I just feel that if someone had pulled Andy over and said he could be whatever he wanted to be, given him that extra bit of confidence, it would have helped him enormously. During Howard's time in charge, you always felt there was an undercurrent between him and Andy, and maybe he lacked a bit of belief because of that. He had ability, fantastic ability, and his left foot could open a tin can. But I just felt that people missed a trick with Andy. Sometimes that is not the player's fault. Sometimes you need the coaches to play their part in getting the best out of someone, to make them believe in themselves.

Anders Limpar:

Anders was maybe the one luxury we had in the team, but we knew he was important for us that day if we were going to pull off a shock. The plan was to get the ball to him as high up the pitch as we could, and let him do his stuff. He had great feet, could go inside and outside, and was technically a very good player. He played very well against United, keeping the ball and giving the rest of us a breather.

Paul Rideout:

'The Cabbage' – I don't know why he was called that, but it stuck – was very under-rated in my opinion. He had a good touch, was decent in the air, could hold up play effectively and he obviously weighed in with the all-important winning goal. Having a Cup final winner's medal is wonderful, but being able to remind the world that you also scored the winning goal is something else. I suppose that must be every striker's dream, and Paul fulfilled that. He was another who I thought could have done more if people had instilled more confidence in him.

Daniel Amokachi (Sub for Limpar, 69 minutes):

He was responsible, along with Nev, for christening me 'Ninja Man' though I never did get to the bottom of that one. You can usually gauge from the first few days of training with someone what they are like, and Daniel had the physique, the pace and the ability to score goals to make him a huge star. He became an enigma, however, and never reached the heights we thought he would. Off the field he was a lovely, lovely lad.

Duncan Ferguson (Sub for Rideout, 51 minutes):

If you asked people to write down what they imagined Duncan to be like, 'easy-going' and 'down-to-earth' probably wouldn't be the first things they'd put. But that is the truth. He wasn't a superstar. He just mucked in with everyone else. I roomed with him before the final and he was just quiet. He made a decent cup of tea and was just normal, not the wild child everyone on the outside made him out to be. All the lads liked a drink back then, but some of us had wives and children and the ones who didn't could stay out a bit longer. If Duncan wanted to stay out, he would stay out but there was never really any trouble because he had good lads looking out for him.

We used to go to the old Retro bar in Mathew Street if we'd had a good win or one of the lads had something to celebrate. People wanted to be in and around Duncan, buying him drinks and being seen with him. It is difficult to turn it down in that situation, but as far as I am concerned he handled it well. I like him a lot and actually introduced him to the woman who would become his wife. A week or so before the Cup final, we were out at some do and John Parrott's sister-in-law, a girl called Janine, asked me to introduce her to Duncan. That was that. They hit it off.

I don't know if it was Duncan's influence, but the post-match party at the Winchester Hotel included a performance from a pipe band while we were eating, the full works. Jacqueline was heavily pregnant at the time so we didn't stay up too late, but a lot of the lads partied until the small hours and then through the next day. We got the coach back to Liverpool and were stopping off at service stations to fill up on drink as much as petrol, before heading off on an open-top bus tour of the city.

It was a different kind of success to that I had enjoyed earlier in my career at the club across the city because it was so unexpected. Because of that, what Everton achieved is up there with anything I did at Liverpool. To be able to say I am the only player who has won FA Cup winners' medals with both Merseyside clubs is massively important to me, and is a slice of football history I don't see being emulated for some considerable time.

The medals are in a box in the loft and don't come out very often. There will come a time when they aren't of use to me anymore and the kids will have to decide whether to sell them or not. I won't mind if they do auction them off because what I achieved is there, written in the history books. I have the memories of those two great days to fall back on. They are as fresh as ever.

* * * * * * * * * * * * * * * * * *

Joe Royle was always keen on us pushing ourselves and not settling for what we had. In that sense, winning the Charity Shield against Blackburn Rovers at Wembley in the curtain raiser to the new season was the perfect response: another trip to Wembley, and another piece of silverware in the trophy cabinet.

Vinny offered a reminder of his talent that day, scoring with a great lob over Tim Flowers to seal our 1-0 success over the champions, but his relationship with the gaffer still meant those days were few and far between. We had European football to look forward to, although our adventure was to prove short-lived. KR Reykjavik had been beaten fairly comfortably over two legs, 6-3 on aggregate, before we were drawn against Feyenoord.

They were always going to be tough opponents and, after drawing 0-0 at Goodison, we lost 1-0 over there thanks to a Regi Blinker goal. That only told half the story, though. We had chances to get the away goal that would have taken us through, and Ronald Koeman was responsible for getting Craig Short sent off as well. Everton had waited so long for European football, and had been denied the chance to compete against the best due to the ban on English clubs after Heysel, so it was a major disappointment to go out so soon. The sense of anti-climax was palpable.

Still, we had high hopes for getting back into Europe again through the league, especially when we signed Andrei Kanchelskis from Manchester United. Andrei took a little while to settle, but when he did he banged them in, finishing the season with 16 goals. He opened his account with two against Liverpool in a 2-1 win at Anfield, which is never a bad way to ingratiate yourself with the supporters, and he never looked back.

However, it wasn't just Liverpool who suffered that day. I went into a challenge with Rushie and damaged my knee ligaments in the process, so had to be helped off by the physio Les Helm. As I made my way down the tunnel, the crescendo of boos around the ground reached deafening levels. That hurt me. Okay, I played for Everton now, but I'd given my all when I had been at Liverpool. I guess I didn't owe them anything and they didn't owe me anything. Maybe it was asking too much for an Everton player, even one who had pulled on a red jersey, to be applauded as they hobbled off, but I don't think I deserved the abuse I received that day.

There had never been any sense from me of "ha ha, you're struggling" when I'd left Liverpool. Graeme had gone on to lose his job, but I took no satisfaction from seeing Manchester United embark on a new era of dominance. Joe was raging afterwards about the reception

I had got, and vowed that he'd never be involved in a transfer that saw a player go between the clubs and, in doing so, left him open to that kind of treatment.

I came back from the injury, but my last game for Everton proved to be an FA Cup fourth-round tie at home to Port Vale in January 1996. Duncan and Daniel scored in a 2-2 draw at Goodison, but my time there had drawn to a close. I just wanted to play. I was 30 and playing reserve-team football for Everton which, at that age, was no good for me. It's not the same as it is now, where you have a squad and you have seven substitutes. It wasn't for me and Joe understood. He couldn't offer me a regular place, and I didn't want to spend my Saturday afternoons watching from the stands.

The club has stayed with me over the years. As I say, I keep in touch with Matt Jackson and Vinny a lot. Whenever I see Howard or hear from him through a friend, Ray Parr, the message is always the same: "Keep going. Keep beating this bloody disease." From Liverpool, Alan Hansen, Jim Beglin and Ronnie Whelan have been in touch to see how my fight against cancer is going. Kenny has called a few times and invited Reece and Riley, my sons, down to watch training. It is nice to know that people are still thinking about you.

But I would have to say the support I have received from Everton has been second to none. I know there has been a tremendous change around in staff at Liverpool since I was there, but it is Everton who have bent over backwards for me, even down to the letters and other correspondence I've received from supporters and so on. If I need training kit for when I'm on my exercise bike, it's no problem. Moyesey will invite me down to watch training at Finch Farm, and the girls in the canteen can't do enough for me.

Bill Kenwright goes way back with my dad and always asks about him before, every time, adding: "How are you, son? If you ever need anything you know where I am. Ring me, I'll always help."

The Everton Former Players' Foundation, thanks to club reverend Harry Ross and Darren Griffiths, who is also the club's press officer, have been fantastic, paying for an exercise bike when I needed one, things like that. They are only ever a phone call away.

In contrast, I got a letter off Liverpool last summer asking if I played golf. They wanted me to take part in some commercial or sponsors' day, where businesses pay to play a round with an ex-Liverpool player. 'Well, I used to play, but right now is not such a good time for me,' I thought as I read it. 'I might struggle for the full 18 holes.'

I made my excuses and sent it back.

People can look at that two ways. I think for a spell before Kenny came back, Liverpool became a colder club because those in charge weren't in touch with how such a great institution was founded. You can say that sending a letter, asking someone who has got cancer if they want to play a round of golf is insensitive and shows they've lost touch.

But I wasn't angry or anything. I didn't see it as a major slight. I just look at that and, well, at least they are thinking of me. I've had invites to the former players' Christmas lunch in the last couple of years as well. It's just whether I am strong enough to attend.

Everton is a fantastic club, run by a fantastic manager who, I hope, eventually gets a little bit of luck in terms of the finance he has to work with. Bill too, for that matter, because what he has done as chairman is not appreciated. I was invited to Everton's Player of the Year awards in 2011 at the King's Dock and I really wanted to say 'thank you' to everyone for their support and kindness, but the excellent Leighton Baines kept on getting award after award. If it wasn't him it was Seamus Coleman, and the night overran.

So now's my chance. David Moyes was right in what he said. Everton is the People's Club.

12

Insult To Injury

When I look back on my career, I recognise I was fortunate to play for two of the biggest clubs in English football. I had the best of everything: I played with the best players, stayed in the best hotels, enjoyed the best times the game could offer anyone. Take a step down the ladder though, and the rungs become rather more treacherous.

Over the course of the season after the FA Cup final success, 1995/96, I slipped down the pecking order under Joe. David Unsworth was playing alongside Waggy in the middle of the defence, and Earl Barrett and Andy Hinchcliffe were considered the first-choice full-backs. Not that I was up in arms to find myself on the fringes of the side. There was no angry fall-out with Joe.

I could have stayed and fought to force my way back into the manager's plans, but in March 1996 an old friend got back in contact: Howard Kendall fancied a reunion. He was in charge of Sheffield United in the Championship and they were struggling badly, embroiled in a relegation fight, and the boss wanted my experience to help get them out of the mess they were in. If it had been any other manager I might have thought twice, but with Howard that was not an issue. I joined them on loan until the end of the season in a flash.

The move was perfect for me. I had missed playing week in, week out, and I would be with a manager who I knew inside out. Not that the move was easy for all of us. My family and I stayed in a hotel for three months, and Scarlet was still just six months old, so that made life very interesting!

She had just started crawling so she would either be off exploring or would whiz round the room in her walker. Luckily it was quite a big room, which meant we could have her cot at one end and still watch the TV in the evening at the other. From what I remember there weren't too many sleepless nights. Some players retire to bed when they come home from training and need lots of sleep to ensure they feel right for the weekend. I've never really been like that, and so the temporary living arrangements never impacted on me in that sense.

Jacqueline had just found out she was pregnant with Reece as well so there was a lot going on, but to begin with, living out of a suitcase was a novelty for us.

We had all our meals done for us, we could go for a swim in the hotel and because I trained for two hours in the morning it meant I was around for the rest of the day to help out. Towards the end of the three months it became more of a bind, but it honestly wasn't as bad as people might think.

United were paying me £4,000 if we won with bonuses and every- thing else, and there would be an extra bonus of £5,000 if we man- aged to stay up. At the end of the campaign, I could then return to Everton and try and prove that I wasn't finished there.

We were two points off the bottom of the division when I went there, but I looked around the dressing room and thought we had a good chance of clawing our way to safety. There were decent players at the club. David White, Mitch Ward, Andy Walker and Michel Vonk were among my new team-mates and, true enough, we embarked on a great run – winning eight, drawing three and losing only one of our final 12 matches – and ended up not finishing too far off the play-offs. That represented some turnaround.

On the final day of the season we were at home to Port Vale and I decided to go and see the chairman, Mike McDonald, because I was due some money. He was the club's third chairman that season alone – a reflection of the turmoil at the place – and had taken over in December and given Howard funds to steady things on the pitch. With my bonus, money for winning a game and a few other bits and bobs, I felt I was owed around £10,000. Yet he went and offered to give me £1,000, and insisted that he couldn't get his hands on any more money there and then.

"That's not right," I said. "There is revenue there from the cash on the turnstiles. We agreed on the figure when I came."

He asked me to leave it with him. But I wasn't happy, and I told Howard that I was keeping the green Rover car the club had given me as a runaround, until the situation got sorted out. Howard asked me if I knew what I was doing, but my attitude was very much along the lines of: 'What's the chairman doing with me?' I felt as if I was being taken for a ride.

I went to the chairman's scrapyard in Manchester a week or two later with my solicitor, Richard Hallows, to see him. I didn't want any trouble. Rather, I just wanted what I felt I was owed. On top of the £1,000 he'd already given me, McDonald then offered me another £3,000. It still fell well short of what I was due. "I'm going on holiday tomorrow and you owe me £6,000," was my response.

The chairman was unimpressed. He made it pretty clear that he wasn't used to people speaking to him like that, but put his hand in his pocket and produced the £3,000. I took it and left. As I headed home, I knew that I'd have to whistle for the rest of the money and, to this day, I am still owed the cash. I suppose he won in the end. I even dropped the car back but, after doing so well for Sheffield United and enjoying playing for the club, it turned the whole episode completely sour for me. Even if Howard had wanted me to sign permanently, there was no way I would have considered it. How could I have worked for a club that had just treated me like that?

As it was, it was another side in the second tier who offered me the chance to keep on playing. While I wanted ideally to go back to Everton and play in the Premier League, there was so much going on in my life off the pitch.

I was in the process of going through a divorce, and they were difficult times. I had split up from my first wife, with whom I had two boys, Josh and Fraser, before I met Jacqueline.

I was building a new life, and moving on caused a lot of upheaval. I suppose it was nothing different to what other people go through when they get divorced, but Joe used to say to me that he didn't know how I managed to go into training with a smile on my face.

So when Birmingham City offered £390,000 for me in June of that year and Everton accepted it, it seemed like a good move. It gave me the opportunity to escape Merseyside for a while, and put some distance between me and all the arguments that were on-going between all the lawyers.

In any case, Birmingham had big ambitions. Though it was a step down from the top flight, I was genuinely excited about the opportunity that awaited me at St Andrew's. The manager, Trevor Francis, was desperate to get into the Premier League and had the support of the board to recruit some top-class, experienced players, who he hoped would help the club make the step up within a couple of seasons.

Steve Bruce had decided to go there from Manchester United, Barry

Horne had moved in the same summer as me and Mike Newell, who I knew from schools football in Liverpool, was leading the line. I didn't know Trevor, Mick Mills or Frank Barlow particularly well, but they were football people and the ideas they outlined to me sounded good. They were trying to build something special. Above them the club's owners, David Sullivan and David Gold, were also eager to kick on.

To be honest, the owners kept themselves to themselves for most of the time I was there. They weren't the type of people who would appear at training every day and get in the ear of the manager.

We once went out as a group, players and wives, to see Jasper Carrott in one of the theatres in Birmingham and they came along, taking us all out for a meal afterwards. But other than that, there wasn't too much contact with them. I always thought I had a fairly decent relationship with them, although having said that I knew they were hard-nosed businessmen – a point that would later be confirmed to me.

There were 50-odd pros on the books when I joined, a legacy of Barry Fry's wheeling and dealing in the preceding period. Among them was Steve Finnan, a youngster at the time whose nomadic journey through the divisions would eventually lead him to Liverpool. But Trevor started weeding out the weaker squad members, trimming round the edges and shaping us into a more manageable group.

He was the sort of manager who wanted to join in training all the time and show the players that he still had the skills that had made him the country's first £1m footballer, and saw him win two European Cups with Nottingham Forest under Brian Clough. The majority of us thought he was like a bar of chocolate: if he could have eaten himself, he would have.

Perhaps it was inevitable that the team took time to bed in and, that first season, we only finished mid-table. I played alongside Brucey initially at the heart of the defence, and what an education that was – even at my age. You could see the class that he had. He would draw forwards under the ball, then collect it on his chest and clip balls nonchalantly up-field to Newelly and Paul Furlong. I really enjoyed our partnership. He was a good player, and you could tell.

Yet Steve actually fell out with Trevor not that long after he arrived and, eventually, I took over as captain. The problem was that the team was constantly evolving. The likes of Dele Adebola, Jon McCarthy and Chris Holland came in and, amid all the chopping and changing, we never quite made it to the Premier League. We finished just outside the play-offs in the second season and then fourth the year after, only to lose to Watford in the play-offs. I watched that game from the sidelines, my season having long since been curtailed plunging my playing career very much in jeopardy.

Maybe it was just age catching up with me, but for some reason I had more injuries at Birmingham than I'd ever had before in my career. I broke my wrist – actually, one of the small bones on the outside of the hand – when a ball struck it in training, and I had to get permission to carry on playing with a cast. The referees were happy enough to allow it, so I would strap up the plaster cast that I already had on but the problem then was co-ordination and balance. When I tried to jump and head the ball, I had what felt like a lead weight on one side of my body dragging me down. I also had an operation to cure a double hernia, although that was nothing compared to what was to follow.

My career effectively ended at Selhurst Park – the ground where my Liverpool career began – on Saturday February 6, 1999, during a game against Crystal Palace. In fact, if you want to be even more precise, it was at 3.22pm that afternoon when everything I had ever worked for was ripped away from me.

The build-up to the match had been been mixed. After living in Solihull for a year, I had moved back to Southport with the family and I used to commute to Birmingham every day from the north-west. I'd drive to Knutsford services and pick up Brucey and then on to Sandbach to pick up Jon McCarthy, and we'd all share the journey from there. At times, the M6 became such a nightmare that I would go by train. I'd catch the 7am rattler from Southport to Liverpool Central, walk from there to Lime Street and then catch the express to Birmingham New Street. The last leg of the daily trek was a taxi to the training ground. You could do it and still be in training by 9.30am, and I used to meet Steve on the train sometimes, too. But it was draining.

The day before the Palace game I had decided to drive to the training ground to catch the team coach, but got caught in traffic on the motorway and, having missed the bus, I had to make my own way down to London. I eventually reached the team hotel and apologised to Trevor. It wasn't the example the captain should be setting, but he was fine about it. These things happen. In fact, he had some good news. We had been in talks over a new contract for a while, and he said the board had agreed to give me another deal which would run until the summer of 2000.

I was relieved, content – even happy. "That's great, thanks a lot," I said, with everything verbally agreed with Trevor. He announced that we'd effectively done a deal to the rest of the team at dinner that night, saying how pleased he was that the captain was staying and how good it was for the team and for what we hoped to achieve.

But my sense of relief barely lasted a day.

I can remember now that the ball was being played down the line midway through the first half, and I moved across to try and clear it. It was a routine situation, nothing particularly risky, but Lee Bradbury hit me from one side and Hayden Mullins from the other. My right knee buckled instantly on impact, and I collapsed to the turf. That was it. I may not have known it at the time, but it was all over.

The strange thing was that when the physio, Neil McDairmid, came running on to treat me, I wasn't writhing around in agony. On the contrary, I couldn't feel anything at all. I was numb. They carried me off on a stretcher and my knee was quickly put in a brace. I knew it was a serious injury, but I had other worries to occupy me in the short-term: like how to get home, for starters. My car was at the team hotel and there was no way I'd be able to drive it – not in that state.

Thankfully, Jon McCarthy volunteered to drive me back to Birmingham. Dele Adebola came along for the ride while I was stretched out on the back seat, but when we got to Birmingham I had to take over. Dele had had his licence taken off him and was banned from driving, so there I was behind the steering wheel with my wobbly knee giving Dele a lift to Liverpool before I drove on to Southport. To this day, I'm still not sure quite how I managed to do that. Maybe the adrenalin was still coursing through my veins. Maybe I was in denial. Somehow, though, I made it back in one piece.

The next day, my dad drove me back down to Birmingham so that I could undergo a series of scans. The news wasn't good. The results came back and the medics couldn't see anything at all in my knee. Nothing. I was told everything had collapsed.

As well as damaging my medial ligaments, I had ruptured my anterior cruciate ligament as well. I was facing at least six months on the sidelines, and maybe another three months or so to get back to match fitness and find some semblance of form. It's not what you want at the age of 33. At least, however, I did have the security of another contract for a year to fall back on. Or so I thought.

When I went into the club on the Monday I was expecting the paperwork to be there for me to sign.

Nothing.

Radio silence.

I probably should have realised what was about to happen. The two Davids and their chief executive, Karren Brady, weren't foolhardy people. They looked to protect the club rather than their skipper.

It was left to Trevor to tell me that the contract wasn't there any more.

It had been withdrawn and, instead, I was being put on a month-to-month deal. I wasn't happy. It wasn't just that I was the captain and thought that I deserved to be treated better. I'd actually agreed everything with the manager verbally on the Friday night. If I hadn't been injured the next day would the contract have still been there? Of course it would. I felt badly let down. There was no big bust-up with Trevor, no ruck. I just let him know I was massively disappointed.

But first things first – I had to concentrate on my rehabilitation. I was told I would need two operations, but the second one, to repair my cruciate, would only take place when I could achieve a 90-degree bend back into the knee. Trying to achieve that goal was agony. Sheer. Bloody. Agony. It is the most pain I have ever felt in my life. I would lie on my front in the gym, Neil would get a wet towel, wrap it round my knee and try and get it to bend.

At first, the other lads used to come in the gym and laugh at me, taking the piss at their stricken captain. But when they saw the tears in my eyes and realised that I wasn't putting anything on, they stayed away and left me to it. Footballers don't like to see what can happen to their team-mates for fear that it could be them the next time they cross the white line.

We got there in the end – goodness knows how because I was ready to give in at times, the pain was so excruciating – and I was told I could have the cruciate operated on. I will always remember I had just had the anaesthetic and was drifting off when the surgeon, Keith Porter – who was brilliant at what he did, and who used to get flown specially into accidents on motorways and serious incidents like that to help out because he was so good – looked up from reading his paper.

"Don't worry, Gary, it'll be fine today." Then he whipped out a black felt tip pen from his pocket and drew a big arrow on my right knee.

The last thought that went through my mind before I went under was: 'Bloody hell. If he has to remind himself which knee it is, maybe

I'm not in such great hands after all.'

As it was, after 124 matches, I never played for Birmingham City again. I eventually came back from the injury but, in the December, I went on loan to Wycombe Wanderers under Lawrie Sanchez and Terry Gibson, two of the players who had starred for Wimbledon against my Liverpool side back in 1988. The fact that I hadn't got close enough to Lawrie for his winning goal at Wembley, thus helping to make him a star, was never mentioned. Wycombe were serious about what they were trying to achieve and I really enjoyed my time there, even though I only played four matches.

My biggest problem was that I was nowhere near the player I had been. The knee still ached, I was in constant pain and, while I could disguise it to an extent in matches, I knew that it wouldn't last. Birmingham knew it, too.

At 5pm on New Year's Eve, 1999, I got a phone call at home from Trevor Francis, asking if I could come down for a chat in the next couple of days. "What's the point, Trevor?" I asked. "I'm not going to come all the way down there just to be told I'm not wanted anymore. That's what you are going to tell me, isn't it?"

"Yes, but I thought this was the right way to do it."

"Don't bother."

That was the last time I spoke to Trevor. In fairness, I haven't run into him since, but he badly let me down over the contract. Nine months after my knee had effectively 'exploded' I had been released by Birmingham City. But my fight with them wasn't over.

They – and I include Sullivan, Gold and Karren as well as Trevor – had given me their word over that new deal and they should have offered me a chance to recover properly, so I consulted the Professional Footballers' Association and took the club to a Football League tribunal. It was not a decision I took lightly, and I am sure I spent more time weighing up what to do than they had in taking the contract off the table, but I felt I had a case.

Brendon Batson and a lawyer from the PFA represented me at a hearing in front of a Football League tribunal in London, while Birmingham had Karren, Trevor and Henri Brandman, who was Gary Glitter's lawyer. We both stated our cases and I was expecting an answer in a couple of weeks. In fact, we had been in recess for only half-an-hour when we were called straight back in. The panel came down on Birmingham's side and said that, because I hadn't signed anything, I had no rights.

I had been warned that this might happen beforehand, but had still thought I had enough on my side to proceed. The lads in the dressing room were on my side. They had sympathy for me because they knew it could be them next. I was gutted.

Afterwards Frank Clark, who had played for Newcastle and won a title and the European Cup with Nottingham Forest, and who had been on the panel, came over to me. "That's a disgrace. If I had been your manager, you would have got two years straight away." He had apparently been out-voted 2-1.

Karren Brady gave me a kiss and said she was sorry that it had to come to this. The Birmingham co-owner David Sullivan was not so kind. When I was released, he publicly said that they had stood by me for nine months, but that there was only "so much you can do."

"It's tough for him but we cannot be the Mr Nice Guy all the time," he added. "Our wage bill has gone ballistic and the gravy train has got to stop."

Mr Nice Guy? I will let other people decide what they think of that.

* * * * * * * * * * * * * * * * * *

After my release from Birmingham, Brian Laws showed some interest in taking me to Scunthorpe United. Indeed, he'd gone as far as to arrange for me to play a game for them one Saturday for the first team, only for Steve McMahon to call me the night before. He was the manager at Blackpool then, in what is now League One, and offered me a six-month contract.

Brian wasn't too happy but I asked him whether Scunthorpe could match it and he said they couldn't, so I headed home and joined up with Blackpool the next day. If I am being honest, I think Steve was doing me a favour. If I hadn't been his team-mate at Liverpool, I'm not sure I would have got the call. But I was grateful for the opportunity and had accepted it because I thought that, the more I trained, the better my knee would be. I was kidding myself. It quickly became clear that wasn't going to be the case.

My debut came in a 1-0 win against Mansfield Town at Field Mill, and I scored on my home debut in a 3-3 draw with Luton Town at Bloomfield Road four days later. But I couldn't run how I wanted, I wasn't pain free and, before too long, Steve left me out of the starting line-up, probably to protect me as much as anything.

As a manager, he was similar in many respects to Graeme Souness: tough, demanding, confrontational, hard-nosed. He was no different to me just because I once shared a dressing room with him as a player. To him, I was just another one of the lads. If he had to chew me out, he did. If I felt a bollocking was just, no problem. Other times, I would argue my point.

My last game in English football came on Saturday, March 11 2000, in a 2-2 draw with Cardiff City in front of 5,015 fans at Bloomfield Road. I came on after 35 minutes as a substitute for John Hills, who had earlier put us 2-0 up from the penalty spot. I had experienced everything from a throbbing Anfield to a bouncing Goodison Park to a packed Wembley over the course of my career. My final game as a player in this country was none of those things.

13

New Life

I loved New York. On Sundays, the whole family would get the train from Baldwin Station on Long Island, where we rented a three-bedroom house, and travel into Penn Station in Manhattan. We'd walk up the stairs, emerging by Madison Square Garden, and the first thing that would hit you was the sheer size of the buildings. Sky scrapers that towered so high they disappeared into the clouds.

There were yellow taxis everywhere, a mass of people cluttering up the sidewalks. It was bedlam – and I used to think it was fantastic. Thrilling. Vibrant. We'd go to Central Park, to the zoo, to Times Square. I remember walking through that neon wonderland with Scarlet on my shoulders once and this fella passed by and, all matter of fact, he said: "Alright, Gary." I did a double take, but he didn't stop. Just carried on walking. It's a small world, sometimes.

We would go to a restaurant called the Olive Garden, or haggle for watches and bags in Chinatown, hoping to get some bargains for friends. The kids loved it, too. Riley was a baby, Reece was in kinder-garten and Scarlet was in school. They both learnt Spanish and, last year, Scarlet passed her GCSE in it. Reece is taking it now. Their dad was never going to be a linguist, but maybe that time spent in the Big Apple gave them an ear for it. We were there for 20 months all in all, and I miss New York. I really do. One of the hardest things about this illness is not allowing yourself to think too far ahead, and I don't know whether I will ever get the chance to go back again. But I really hope that I can.

The opportunity to relocate there had come about through a lad called Paul Riley, who I had gone to school with. He hadn't been a bad player in his own right and played for Liverpool Schoolboys. I sort of kept in touch with him and he had set up his own company, Paul Riley Soccer Schools, and was head coach of the team, Long Island Rough Riders.

"Why don't you come over," he had said. "You'll like it, and the foot-ball will suit you now."

I discussed it with Jacqueline and decided I would give it a go. I went for six weeks on my own, doing some coaching and playing for the Rough Riders, probably earning more money than any of the other players. The Long Island Ducks were a baseball team and we occa-sionally played at their stadium in front of crowds of around 3,000-4,000. The standard was okay. To offer a comparison with the English leagues, I would say that we would have struggled to hold our own in League One, but we would have been comfortable in League Two.

Importantly for me on a personal level, my knee was standing up to it. I played in central midfield and would just get it and pass it. We played in a midfield three, so I had two others to do my running if needs be anyway.

I was enjoying the whole experience and so persuaded Jacqueline that this was something we should try together. It was a nice standard of life, if a little expensive, but I thought we should give it a try. We lived with Paul in his house, initially. Then, we got our own place in Nile Street in a village called Ocean Side. I would train in the morning, have the afternoon together with Jacqueline and the kids, and then go off and train various teams at night.

The appetite for football in America surprised me: it's huge. We tend to have a patronising view of football there in England. But, up until the age of 18, it is as big in the United States as it is anywhere in the world. After that, admittedly, it loses its thread because people go to college until they are 22 and, by the time they come out, their outlook has changed. But I recognised that this was a wonderful opportunity to get involved in the sport over there.

Paul ran a team called Albertson, which was a really rich Jewish club, and I coached the Under-12s and Under-13s. When the parents of the kids had pool parties and barbeques, we would all be invited. It was brilliant. It wasn't like a job. From that I got work all over Long Island and would do a couple of hours of coaching a night. Yet, for some reason, it turned sour.

I don't know whether Paul thought I was getting too big for my boots. I was keen to get involved, keen to do this and that, and maybe he thought I was trying to push him to the side. As a result, the relationship we had deteriorated rapidly to the point where we hardly spoke to one another. Or, if we did, it was only when we absolutely had to. We both went about our business, but we were sadly becoming rivals rather than friends.

Things changed on the pitch, too. The Rough Riders won the Northeast Division in 2000 but lost in the play-offs, and the next season proved disastrous. We finished 42 points behind divisional champions, Hershey Wildcats, and out of the play-offs. The club's owners voluntarily relegated the team to D3 Pro League for the following season.

I think money worries played a part in the decision – travel costs alone must have been exorbitant. We could play against Rochester, who were 11 hours away on a bus, but we would still be in New York State. That is how far the league spanned.

Paul said he didn't think I should be playing at this standard any more, and I wasn't afforded the opportunity to re-sign and play like some of the other lads, probably because I was on more money than any of them. We ended up falling out and not speaking to each other. Things got petty between us.

I suppose it didn't help that another coach, Mick McDermott, had approached me about taking over the running of Albertson. Mick, who went on to work as Carlos Queiroz's fitness coach with the Iran national team, had arranged a meeting with Gerard Terry, who was the chairman of the club, in a deli. He was prepared to plough $500,000 into the club, paying for everything from the coaching staff to the hiring of pitches, and we outlined our plan to him. There was a lot to do. Albertson runs teams from Under-4s to Under-18s, for boys, girls and also mixed sides. This was a major project.

A board meeting was called in a diner. We stated our case, Paul stated his in a separate meeting. In the end, they opted to go with Paul. He is now the director of coaching at the Albertson Academy, and the set-up is doing really well. Fair play to him – he's done well over there – but our own American Dream eventually ended in February 2002. But it wasn't just football that played a part in our decision to return home.

September 11, 2001. Recognise that date? We had just dropped the kids off at school that morning when a mother of one of the boys in Reece's class said a plane had flown into the World Trade Centre. Like everyone else, we were shocked, but thought it must have been some kind of terrible accident. On the way back home, Jacqueline and I stopped off to get a cup of tea and it was then that the news came over that a second plane had hit the towers. So this was no accident at all.

The sense at the time was one of panic. You worried that the terrorist atrocity, which was clearly what it was, would start a chain of events and that the world was going to end. The first thing we did was to go and get the kids from school and head home. I just sat transfixed in front of the television watching in disbelief. In England, we've sort of grown accustomed over the years to bombs and attacks with the IRA, but this was relatively unheard of in the USA.

A lot of people in the area we lived in lost relatives that day, and there were candlelight vigils in our neighbourhood. The eeriness of it all struck you. We lived on the flight path to JFK and, when all the planes were grounded, the silence struck you because we were used to the distant roar of the jet engines above. Every few minutes there would usually be planes whizzing overhead, either coming in to land or taking off. Yet, for days afterwards, if you heard the sound of a jet it was probably a fighter guarding the skies.

New York changed. Instead of the vibrant city we all had come to love, there was a nervousness about the place, which was a huge shame but totally understandable in the tragic circumstances. The concern that the events of 9/11 might repeat themselves was part of our decision to come home. My mum used to come over, as did Jacqueline's mum, but after the attack they stopped. Naturally, they worried about us, worried about their grandkids and they wanted us to come home.

We might have been ready to return by then, anyway. I had sensed the writing was on the wall for a while, and had started writing to clubs in England asking whether they had any coaching positions available that I might fill. Liverpool said 'no, but thanks'. I got a nice letter back from Arsene Wenger, also saying there was nothing at the moment.

It wasn't just the big clubs, either. I wrote across the board, and was actually asked to go on trial by Grimsby Town as a player. I was 36 at the time, my knee was still playing up, but their manager, Paul Groves, pleaded with me to go. I went over but always knew an unlikely resumption of my professional career was never really going to happen.

The intensity of the training and practice matches was too much. My knee was too sore, and I spent the evenings while I was there wondering what I was going to do with myself.

In the end, I got lucky. We were staying at Jacqueline's mum's house in City Road, right in the shadow of Goodison Park, when we came back from the USA. Everton's youth team were playing against Nottingham Forest in an FA Youth Cup tie, so I decided to pop across and take a look. In actual fact, it was more a case of Wayne Rooney versus Michael Dawson that night. Wayne came out on top, scoring in a 2-1 victory, and Everton reached the final that year before losing to a strong Aston Villa side.

Wayne was only 16, but you could see he was going to be a superstar. He was strong, but it was his game intelligence that set him apart. He knew instinctively what to do when the ball came to him, and where to be on the pitch in order to cause the most havoc. He ran the show, as he has done for every side he's played for in the years since.

I bumped into Ray Hall, Everton's academy director at the game, as well as Neil Dewsnip, head coach, and Mike Dickinson, who is the club's education welfare officer, and we got talking. One of Everton's coaches, David Lowe, was moving to a new job at the PFA and they asked me to come in for a chat the next day. I met them and they offered me a coaching role there and then. There was an opportunity to take one of the age groups on, and then do as much coaching as I wanted at night.

Everton paid £30-a-session and I did three sessions a night, four nights a week. I also worked Saturday and Sunday. The age groups I was assigned to were 12 to 16-year-olds and, while it was hard work, it was a good chance to take my first steps into coaching in England. It was a great opportunity. Just what I needed.

Mike fast-tracked me on a coaching course at Keele University so that I could do my badges. Paul Ince was enrolled on the same one, but he went on holiday half-way through it. Peter Schmeichel was another. He used to turn up in his flip-flops and with a packet of cigarettes, and he just struck me as not being interested. Why bother if that's your attitude? It was a two-week, intensive training course, and I enjoyed it. You are taught how to put on training sessions, with the emphasis always on progress – getting the kids to progress. Then when I returned to Everton, Andy Barlow, the ex-Oldham player who by then was an FA assessor, oversaw what I was doing and passed me.

When Colin Harvey left, I was moved up along with some of the other coaches and took over the Under-17s, who were based at Netherton in the north of Liverpool, not too far away from Aintree Racecourse. We had steady players, the likes of Mark Hughes and Laurence Wilson – Mark's at Bury now and Laurence at Morecambe – and we reached the National Finals in 2004, but we ran into an Aston Villa side that was just too strong. They had the Moore brothers, Stefan and Luke, Craig Gardner and Gabriel Agbonlahor, and ran away with it. They beat us 5-1 at Villa Park before we salvaged a bit of pride at Goodison Park a week later when we drew 1-1. There was no shame in losing the final to them.

We took the youngsters to an army base in Brimstone in Devon one pre-season because we were looking for elite performers, and felt the army were the best in that field. We wanted to see if the cocky lads were still as sure of themselves at the end of the course, and whether the exercises they did brought through any unexpected leaders.

Victor Anichebe and James Vaughan were among that group and we had a smashing time. As staff we were told to take a back seat for the three days we were there and not to get involved. We were stationed in the Officers' Mess. We could watch what was going on, but on no account could we interfere.

The lads were treated as proper army cadets, woken up at the crack of dawn and ordered to go on zip slides and assault courses. They dragged each other through tunnels filled with water and discovered a different slant to the concept of team-work. There is a special picture of them all sat in mud, thumbs up for the camera, that hangs in Finch Farm, and I suppose one of the successes of the trip was measured by the fact the officers said they would have taken seven of the players for the Royal Marines straight away.

It was a great experience for all of us, and we made some good friends in the short space of time we were there. Sadly one of the course leaders, Corporal Ben Nowak, who was an Evertonian through and through and was absolutely brilliant with the lads, was later killed in action in Iraq.

As a coach, I was developing my own style. I'd try to put an arm around players and help them as much as I could. I wanted them to know I was on their side. After one reserve game, which had pitted Victor and Vaughany against the experienced Wolves defender Jody Craddock, we had a chat about making life difficult for defenders. The lads were only 16 and said Craddock kept coming out of nowhere to take the ball off them. So we worked on changing one or two things in their game in the hope that it would give them a better awareness of what was happening on the pitch. I always thought that if you give Victor balls in the right areas, balls to his feet on the edge of the box so he can twist and turn, then you've got a hell of a player on your hands. He just needs a few goals to make him believe in himself more. He scored a good poacher's strike against Sheffield United in the League Cup in 2011, but we need to see a bit more of that from him. He needs to get into the box more rather than hanging outside it, not wanting to get hurt.

Everton has to take its academy set-up seriously because of the financial realities that the club has been operating within and, until that changes, the emphasis placed upon the youth system to churn out players will only increase. The only problem is you won't get a Wayne

Rooney or a Ross Barkley coming through every year, demanding everyone sits up and takes notice.

'Mollycoddled' is how I would describe today's kids. The sergeant major regime that I had when I was growing up at 16, 17, 18 never did me any harm. Sweeping changing rooms didn't stunt my development – it actually enhanced it, because it made me appreciate what I had and drummed a sense of respect into me. I learned the hard way. These days, the youngsters are cosseted away from reality. If you go to say something to a teenager today, you will have someone down your throat saying that's not how to talk to them. Everything has become too politically correct.

I would get angry and frustrated at Netherton. The lads would get there for 9am for breakfast, but then wouldn't go out on the pitch until the last minute when training officially started at 10am. They'd sit in the changing room, chatting, messing about, having banter. Not many, if any, got a ball, went out early and practised their passing, sharpened their skills, or even tried out things like different free-kicks.

Do you think David Beckham spent 45 minutes joking in the dressing room when he was 17, or did he spend every available minute on the training ground? Practising, practising, practising. What about Cristiano Ronaldo? Or Lionel Messi? I used to wonder why our lads weren't doing more to improve themselves whenever they could.

Not so long ago I went to see Alan Irvine, who is now academy manager at Everton after his spells in charge of Preston North End and Sheffield Wednesday, and he feels the same. Alan's a great coach and he'll help any youngster at Everton. He'll listen to him, give him his time, offer him his advice, anything he wants. But the kids have to want to do it as well. They have to give him something back. They have to push themselves.

My frustration with them was compounded by my own situation. I wanted to kick-on, but Moyesy had his backroom team in place and I had to respect that. I didn't have much to do with him back then. He had more important things to do than worrying about the coach of the Under-17s, so when you think what he did for me when I was in hospital, coming to visit out of the blue like that when he had no real need to, it serves as a measure of the man.

But, back then, I was ambitious and determined to work higher up the coaching ladder. Soon I found the lure of a familiar destination too hard to resist.

14

Rafa's Team

Every now and again my mobile phone will buzz and a text message will ping through. 'Gary, how are you? Hope everything is okay. Rafa.' I'll read it, punch in a little update on how my recovery is going and text back my reply. But, rather than that proving to be the prelude to a dialogue, nothing will come back.

Two months down the line another text will appear from Rafa Benitez, again just checking how I am. I'll text back. Nothing will come back in return.

It is nice to know that he is still interested in my welfare, that means something to me. Football is what it is. Relationships are forged and are broken just as quickly. Rafa didn't need to send those texts. Plenty of other people my career overlapped didn't. But, if I'm being honest, the lack of interaction rarely comes as much of a surprise to me. When I was sacked by Liverpool in 2009 after three years as reserve-team manager, I never really knew what Rafa was thinking, either. My departure still confuses me to this day.

Rafa is without doubt one of the best coaches that I have ever worked for or with. His attention to detail is amazing, and his knowledge of tactics immense. Yet, from getting on well with him initially, our relationship disintegrated and, within six months of being told I was doing a good job, I was out of the door. As with my playing career at Anfield, my refusal simply to fall into line and be one of the gang probably counted against me.

The prospect of returning to Liverpool had come about by chance. I bumped into Colin Wood, the former Daily Mail journalist who lives not far from me, and someone I knew well from my playing days, in the village one afternoon. He mentioned that Liverpool were looking for a new reserve coach. Paco Herrera, whom Rafa had brought over from Spain, wanted to go back home and take up a job with Espanyol and the position was up for grabs.

I was anxious to get on in my career, but knew that the opportunities to progress were always going to be limited at Everton because David Moyes already had a structure in place which he trusted and was comfortable with. That was fair enough. But, in the circumstances, the opportunity to work up the road at Liverpool seemed like too good a chance to pass up.

I managed to get hold of the fax number for Melwood and sent off my CV. I didn't hear anything back so I tried again, this time having acquired Rafa's private fax number. 'Dear Rafa, I hope you are well. I understand there could be a vacancy in your backroom staff and was hoping you would consider me for the position,' was along the lines of what I sent. Again, I heard nothing back.

Then, a few days later, I was doing the weekly shop at Asda when my mobile rang. There was a Spanish voice on the other end and I immediately thought: 'Who's this taking the piss?' The thing was, not many people knew I had applied for the job. Certainly no one did at Everton, where I was still working, so I played along for a few seconds before it dawned on me properly that this wasn't a joke.

"It's Rafa Benitez. Would you be interested in coming in for an interview for the reserve job?"

This was genuine. "Of course, Rafa. When?"

"This afternoon?"

I lashed the trolley to one side in the aisle, leaving all the shopping stacked up in it, and rushed home to have a shave and get suited and booted. The drive to Melwood took about half-an-hour. I was thinking about all the things I was going to say and trying to imagine what he would ask me, rehearsing in my mind how things would play out. I knew how much of an opportunity this was, and I couldn't afford not to take it. The chance of working at Liverpool doesn't come around too often, for anyone.

As it was, I had another half-an-hour to wait and compose myself upon my arrival at the training ground as Rafa finished off some meetings and then called me into his office. There was a bit of chit-chat, but we quickly got down to the nitty gritty, with Rafa quizzing me on his tactics board for an hour. He'd set different scenes and scenarios and asked me what I would do next. Such as: 'The opposition have the ball, where would you squeeze them on the pitch to try and win it back?' Or: 'My team had the ball now, but how would I attack and try and exploit weaknesses in the opposition?' It was full on stuff, but I really enjoyed it.

He took me on a guided tour of Melwood, which had been revamped in recent times, and said he would be back in touch. The wait was torture. A few weeks went by and I had heard nothing, so I called Frank McParland, who was chief scout then but who is now the academy director, to see what was happening. I really wanted the job. It was a chance to progress and, from that first meeting with Rafa, I knew I would be working under someone who was one of the best coaches in

Europe. His knowledge was fantastic.

Liverpool had won the FA Cup in that summer of 2006, a trophy to go alongside the Champions League which had been secured so dramatically the year before in Istanbul, triumphs that ensured Rafa became the first Liverpool manager to win major honours in each of his first two seasons. As far as the fans were concerned you could stick Jose Mourinho, who was making waves down at Chelsea at the time after back-to-back Premier League titles. To them, it was Rafa who was the 'Special One.'

Still, there was nothing official from the club or Frank and, in the meantime, I had been asked by Wycombe Wanderers to go for an interview for the vacant manager's job. I explained to them that I had been interviewed for the post at Liverpool and was waiting for a reply, and they were brilliant about it. They just told me to get back in touch when I knew what I was doing. In the end, Paul Lambert got the job and it proved an excellent stepping stone for him if you see how well he's done since with Norwich City.

But I was getting increasingly anxious. I phoned Frank back and said I needed an answer. The response, when it came, was another test. Rafa got back in touch and asked me to do a presentation on how I saw the season progressing for the reserve team on a piece of paper. "Just one sheet will be fine," he said. "I don't want anything more."

My view was that this could be my one and only chance to get a job at Liverpool, the club where it had all begun for me all those years before. To simply write my thoughts down on what would be the equivalent of the back of a beer mat seemed stupid. With the help of one of my mates, I wrote up a seven-page dossier with graphs and everything, printed it off on the computer and took it down the following day to give it to Rafa.

"What happened to supplying one page?" he said with a smile.

"Rafa, this is my chance to impress you. I'm not going to cut any corners now and worry about what I should have done later."

We went through the presentation for about an hour. It included a physical, mental and lifestyle programme aimed at getting the best out of the lads on the training pitch. Everything seemed to go quite well, although there was another interminable wait for a response. "This is painful this, mate," I said in another phonecall to Frank. I didn't really know him that well, certainly not well enough to keep pestering him as I did. But, eventually, Rafa called me into Melwood and said there was something he wanted to discuss with me.

Surely he wouldn't be dragging me all the way down to Melwood to tell me I'd missed out on the job? "You'd just say that on the phone, wouldn't you, if that was the case?" I said to Jacqueline.

He was seeing some agents and players when I first got there and, for 45 minutes, I was sat with the pot plants in reception, my tie having gone skew-whiff and the top button on my shirt ripped open as I fretted on what the next few minutes would hold for me. Rafa appeared at the top of the stairs and beckoned me up. I went into his office.

"The job is yours," he said. I could have hugged him, but I just rang home instead. I was hysterical, Jacqueline was hysterical. This was everything I had wanted – a chance to work with one of the masters, back at the club I had graced as a player. I had come home.

* * * * * * * * * * * * * * * * *

The hardest part of leaving Liverpool was that, for two years, I had loved the job Rafa Benitez had given me. We also enjoyed such good times as well. That just made my second departure from the club all the more disappointing.

It was pre-season when I joined and, for the first couple of weeks, all I did was shadow Rafa. I grabbed a pen and paper, ready to take notes and pick up any pointers from him, but he told me to put them down.

"No. All we do is repetition," he told me. "You will get it. Don't worry. If I have something to say, I'll say it. If you have a question, ask it."

He was brilliant, to be fair, and by being that close to him I saw how important the smallest little detail is at the highest level. The attention to detail is staggering. Training was very good and fresh, innovative even, and I liked the sessions his assistant, Pako Ayesteran, put on. There were lots of patterns of play, with all of the emphasis placed on retaining possession. Keep the ball, no matter what.

I had been there for two weeks when Rafa gave me a DVD of Real Madrid's B team and asked me to watch it and tell him who the best player was. The player who stood out, head and shoulders above everyone else on the pitch, was a young Juan Mata. He was in the B team at the Bernabéu before eventually going on to make his name at Valencia. When you see the progress he has made since, and the performances he has put in at Chelsea since moving to the Premier League, it seems strange that Liverpool did not take a chance on him there and then, given they were aware he had the potential to be special. Rafa agreed with my assessment and we spoke about the way Mata always seemed to find space and choose the right option. It wasn't much of a test I suppose, because no one else came close to measuring up to him – but it was one I passed all the same.

I was also handed a DVD of a match between Everton and Blackburn Rovers and was asked how I would combat Moyesy's side. Liverpool were due to play them in the Merseyside derby a few weeks from then, and I thought the timing of asking me to watch the tape was interesting. Was this a test from Rafa? After all, I had been on the inside, so to speak, across Stanley Park before arriving back at Liverpool. If it was his way of scrutinising me, I didn't mind. I scribbled down a few notes and, presumably, I passed because a few days later he said he was sending me on a scouting mission to watch PSV Eindhoven against Willem II over in Holland.

Brilliant, this was just what I wanted: the chance to get involved more and show what I could do. PSV were in Liverpool's Champions League group so there was a lot riding on the report I sent back. I knew I couldn't make any mistakes if I didn't want a black mark against my name.

The club sent a car to my house to pick me up, and I was whisked to Liverpool airport to fly to Amsterdam before staying overnight. I caught the train up to where Willem played in Tilburg, and had dinner with one of Frank McParland's mates. It was smashing the way the whole trip was done. I'd never experienced anything like this before. So slick and professional.

PSV won the game 3-1 and I sat there scribbling notes in the directors' box: the team formation; who took the corners and the free-kicks; the substitutes who were used; there was even a penalty so I noted down which way he put it past the goalkeeper. I got home on the Sunday and wrote up the notes for Rafa, before handing them over to him on the Monday morning. I felt I'd done a decent job, and the stuff I'd found out would benefit the side.

The first team was flying to Eindhoven later that morning and, about half-an-hour after I'd seen Rafa, I got a phone call from him. "Gary, I've left the notes on my desk," he said. "Can you find a secure line and fax it through to the hotel? I don't want anyone else to see it."

I figured he must have been pleased with my assessment if he wanted the notes sent to the hotel. As it was, Liverpool drew 0-0 and the game passed by without any real incident, save for Steven Gerrard hitting the bar late on after coming on as a substitute. But it had still been great to be involved. I felt part of the coaching side, a member of the team. I could contribute, even if I knew my main responsibility was with the reserves, and Rafa was clear that he would run the first team. There wasn't going to be much crossover.

That suited me to be honest. I had to do match reports for Rafa on who played, who did well, who to keep an eye on and what the opposition were like, but I basically got on with running the reserves with Ian Sylvester, who was the club's secretary at the time.

My first game in charge of the reserves was a 1-0 defeat to Manchester City, before we got battered 4-1 by Newcastle United. We were taken apart, in all honesty. Afterwards, I was worried. This wasn't the sort of impression that I had wanted to make. But, to Rafa's credit, he called me into his office and just said not to worry about the score, to just be positive and keep pushing the players. It was reassuring, at that point in our relationship, to have a manager who offered that backing and who also had an understanding of the problems I faced.

When I played for Liverpool reserves at the start of my career we would invariably win the title, but that was because we had a lot of homegrown players who knew what was expected of them. Yet, by the time I returned to Melwood, the influx of foreign youngsters into the club had created a clash of cultures. You had to worry about boys settling in, getting them used to things like the food and speaking English. It took a while for them to make that adjustment, and that first season for me, 2006/07, was very much a settling in period into the demands of the role.

There was also the issue of integrating senior players into the set-up. Lots of them were involved that campaign. I used 38 players in all, and the likes of Robbie Fowler, Javier Mascherano, Fabio Aurelio, Alvaro Arbeloa, Harry Kewell, Bolo Zenden and Jermaine Pennant appeared on occasions for the second string. I would work with my players, the younger ones, on a daily basis and hand the team I wanted to play to Rafa. He might, understandably, then say he needed one of the seniors to get a game, and the preparations we had spent the week doing would be disrupted. Well, out of the window, effectively. But that was simply part of the job.

Those senior lads probably didn't want to be there, if truth be told, but I could never fault their attitude. I just used to say to them to go out and try your best for yourselves, and for the lads trying to make their way. I wanted them to set an example, and they did that. For one game against Blackburn Rovers we had about seven seniors in the team, and they were top-class. We won comfortably and Robbie scored a little curler with his left foot, turning his shot into the opposite corner to which the ball came into him. Brilliant – what a player he was.

Other than when they were playing for us, the first-team lads didn't show much interest in the reserves, though that is normal throughout football I suppose. Craig Bellamy joined that same summer and, to his credit, he said that if I needed anything, he would come over and work with the reserves and pass on a few tips. But we started training half-an-hour after the first team and, when Craig was doing his warm down, we would be wrapped up in a practice match so it was difficult to get his input in the end. I appreciated the offer, though.

It was all a huge learning curve for me. To offer an insight into the level of detail that was involved, Rafa had brought over a Spanish planning professor when I was just starting out in the job. He organised the training sessions initially, and the emphasis was always on progression. The lads warmed-up and then would step things up a little bit more in the first stage of training. In all there were four stages, and the last would be something like an eight-a-side game.

Myself and Hughie McAuley watched and learned for a fortnight and put it into practice ourselves, ensuring that theme of progression was maintained throughout our own sessions. It was good and I hadn't seen that before. This all felt innovative, something to give Liverpool an edge over the rest.

If the results weren't particularly eye-catching, then we did make some progress. For example, Jay Spearing was playing at centre-half when he came up to the reserves from the youth ranks, but it was clear that role was never going to be his position if he was going to make the breakthrough. He was too small for central defence, and wasn't cut out to play there. Rafa and I thought that he could do a job at full-back but, really, the position we felt he could flourish in was central midfield so he was switched there.

One of his first games for the reserves was against Manchester United. Lucas Leiva produced a little back heel and Jay clipped it into the corner of the net. It was a nice goal and, from then on, he was always going to play there. He never looked back, and it's great to see him in and around the first team now, showing that there are still local lads who can make it. Jay has a great attitude. He appreciates what he has and those around him, and that makes him something of a rarity in terms of the youngsters coming into football these days. It's not about, 'How much are you going to pay me?' with Jay. He's more the sort who just wants to play. It is no surprise to me that with that attitude he is getting more and more games under Kenny's management. He has matured of course, and is more valuable to the manager now. But his selfless approach is also something the other youngsters coming through the ranks should look at. Jay is a player intent on getting the last drop out of his talent, and what player cannot learn from that?

It was rare for the senior lads to play much for the reserves in the second year. We faced United again and Harry Kewell and Xabi Alonso played in a 2-0 win, but more often than not the group was much younger and more settled, and we were better off for that. We had moved from Wrexham's Racecourse Ground, which we felt was too far away, to Warrington. That was fine, until the rugby league season kicked in and the pitch started to cut up more due to the amount of sport being played on it. By then, however, we were well on the way to topping the table.

Liverpool's reserve team lost just once in 18 matches in the 2007/08 league season – ironically at home to Roy Keane's Sunderland, who had packed their team with senior players – and we conceded just eight goals in all our matches. We had a good team: lads like Jay, Stephen Darby, Mikel San Jose, Ronald Huth, Emiliano Insua, Damien Plessis, Nabil El Zhar, Martin Kelly, Krisztian Nemeth and Dani Pacheco. Nemeth scored 11 goals, Dani got a few and we were tough to play against.

I tried to get us to take the ball down and play as much as we could on the turf, because I felt we had the players to do that well. Training used to focus on passing, patterns of play and getting narrow when we lost possession, and there was a lot of input from Angel Vales, who was someone Rafa had been at university with and had brought over to add to his technical staff. He was very much into the analytical aspects of the game – the timing of sessions, how big the pitches were we played on, those sort of things.

By virtue of finishing top of our table, we reached the National Final and faced Aston Villa in a one-off game that would be played at Anfield. There was bad blood between the clubs at the time. Rafa had targeted Gareth Barry as a potential summer signing and Martin O'Neill had reacted furiously in the media, effectively accusing Liverpool of tapping Barry up and trying to unsettle his player. It added an extra edge to our game, and perhaps explained why Villa fielded such a strong side.

Marlon Harewood and Shaun Maloney were in attack – both seven-figure signings – and Wayne Routledge also lined up for Kevin MacDonald's side. Youngsters like Chris Herd, Barry Bannan and Marc Albrighton also featured. I knew Kevin a little bit from my time as a player at Anfield, but didn't speak to him too much before the game. I just did a bit in the programme that was brought out for the match, to say how well he was doing at Villa.

My team was more or less the same as usual. Jay had injured himself in a game against Accrington Stanley in the Lancashire Senior Cup semi-final and missed out, and Rafa asked Lucas if he would play. We got off to a great start with Nemeth scoring after 11 minutes before Villa came back really strongly. For 20 minutes at the start of the second half, they battered us. You could tell how much they wanted to win by the fact that Martin actually left his seat in the directors' box to be more involved. He had been sitting at the polar opposite end of the row to Rafa, but came down to the touchline at one point and started coaching Kevin's team.

However, we weathered the storm and Jordi Brouwer scored a second midway through the half before Lucas wrapped things up with 13 minutes to go. He was great that night, and showed a really good attitude. I won't try and pretend that the feeling I had that night was the same as winning a league championship or an FA Cup, but I did take a huge amount of pride from seeing us beat Villa and be crowned national champions. The success wasn't all down to me, by any means. No one person ever wins titles. But I took a great deal of personal satisfaction from the way we played that season.

Liverpool, as a club, made the most of the triumph, portraying it as proof that things were looking up at youth level after what had been perceived to have been a barren period.

Things certainly felt as if they were progressing. We went to the Dallas Cup in the United States that Easter and smashed everyone in sight, to the extent that the club hasn't been invited back since.

It was in Dallas that I got to properly meet Tom Hicks, Liverpool's co-owner, for the first time. My impressions of him will not find favour with a lot of supporters, but to me he wasn't the brash, hard-headed, arrogant man that he has been portrayed as. Tom obviously made plenty of enemies during his tumultuous time in charge with George Gillett, but I have to say that the way he and his son, Tommy Jnr, looked after us over there was unbelievable.

You take people as you find them and Tom was cutting short his holiday to come and see us play, turning up in a battered Liverpool shirt and desert wellies, and bent over backwards for us. "Whatever you need, we can provide," he told me. "You can have our own private doctor if there are any problems with any of the lads. Just get in touch if you need to."

He laid on a private box at the American Airlines Center for the team to watch the Dallas Stars ice hockey team, and then provided a meal for everyone. I was a bit cheeky and asked afterwards whether there was any chance of watching the Dallas Mavericks play the Boston Celtics in an NBA match the next night and, again, he couldn't have done more. "No problem," he said and we had the use of his personal box with food laid on.

He eventually resumed his holiday, but returned again when we got to the final of the Dallas Cup and beat the Argentinean side, Tigres, 3-0. I got the feeling that he was someone who was proud to own Liverpool, even if his relationship with the club turned sour in the period that followed. It was obvious that he had money, but patently not the sort of wealth at his immediate disposal that Liverpool needed at that time to over-ride the economic downturn and get on with climbing the ladder back to the top.

We would go on to lose to Manchester United 3-2 in the Lancashire Senior Cup final that year as well, so we could technically have made it a domestic 'double.' That game was played at Leyland the following pre-season because the two clubs' schedules meant it couldn't be fitted in any earlier. By then, however, my time at Liverpool had taken a turn for the worse. It would not be long before I felt completely used.

15

All Change

Rafa told me he was bringing in some new young players in the summer of 2008, and that they would add quality to the squad that had just won the league. Great, I thought, this is how it used to be at Liverpool. No standing still. Everything was a constant attempt to build on success, staying one step ahead of the others.

Then Vitor Flora, Vincent Weijl and Emmanuel Mendy all arrived for small fees. Straight away I didn't think they were on a par with the level of the players we already had.

That would not have been a problem as such, except for the fact that Rafa told me he wanted me to pick these players ahead of others in the squad. I thought there were better local lads available, but it was clear that these three had to take preference. Rafa will deny that, but that is what I took from our conversation.

There would have been coaches who would have done as the manager said and not worried about it, but that isn't the way I am. In my view, none of the players Rafa had brought in on the advice of chief scout Eduardo Macia were good enough to play and I wasn't going to just go along with that, say nothing and watch the team and my coaching career suffer as a result.

Things soon came to a head. Sammy Lee had also returned to Liverpool that summer after spending some time out of the game following his sacking as Bolton Wanderers' manager. He had replaced Alex Miller, who had left to take up a manager's job with JEF United Ichihara Chiba in Japan's J-League. When Alex had made it known he had decided to move on as first-team coach, I went to see Rafa and asked about the vacancy, stressing that I would love the opportunity to step up and work alongside him and the first team.

"I have been thinking about that, but I am thinking of offering Sammy the job," said Rafa. "Anyway, in terms of what you offer with the reserves, you are far more important to me there, building that relationship with them." I was disappointed but, at the same time, I could swallow that. Rafa had said I was doing well. I had clearly made a good impression on him.

As it was, Sammy became the link in many ways between the reserves and the first team. We didn't attend Rafa's meetings in the morning but I would speak, along with the doctors and physio, to Sammy about who was fit and whether the first team needed anyone to join in a session with them. He would go off and liaise with Rafa, and then let us know what was required.

I told Sammy that I felt Vitor, Vincent and Emmanuel weren't going to improve the team. I felt that I'd always had a decent relationship with Sammy, and I told him that in confidence. But Rafa found out and given that Sammy was the only one who knew how I really thought, it figured to me that he had told Rafa. I was disappointed with that. I felt badly let down. I spoke to Sammy, but that was it between us from that point on. The trust had gone. I suppose that, rightly or wrongly, I was questioning his integrity, basically accusing him of being a liar, but who else could have told Rafa?

The situation led to Rafa calling both of us into his office. He never really took anyone's side, and simply said: "I don't want problems. I want solutions. Find them for me." That was it.

But looking back, the fact I would speak up for myself is probably the biggest reason why I left. Maybe Rafa was expecting to get a 'yes man' when he recruited me. Gary McAllister and John Barnes had been linked with the role as well, so it was not as if he was without options. Maybe he thought that with Gary's stock still so high after the treble cup-winning season in 2001, and with Barnesy's place in the club's history forever assured, they would have too much power. But there was no way I was just going to fall in line if I thought Liverpool Football Club could benefit from doing something differently.

The academy and the first team at Liverpool had always enjoyed an unusual relationship. Steve Heighway, the former academy director, did not really get on with Gerard Houllier, the previous manager, and there had been a clash of personalities between him and Rafa as well. It was as if two clubs were operating under the same roof. The lack of crossover was a problem, and I had tried to build a link between the reserves and the academy by bringing players up to train at Melwood. It worked for a while. Rafa would come out and watch, and see who was coming through.

But it probably broke down over Nathan Eccleston. I got my knuckles wrapped for bringing him up to Melwood and, after that, we couldn't really have a decent meeting. I just thought he was better than Vitor. I didn't tell Rafa I was doing it, because we were essentially operating separately and independently. It was my decision to bring him up. But when Rafa found out, he ordered me to send him back to Kirkby, where the academy was based.

I carried the can for trying to integrate him into the reserve team set-up without the manager's green light, and then had to go and tell Nathan that there had been a mistake and that he wouldn't be reporting to Melwood after all. He was obviously very disappointed – and he had every right to be.

Add that to the undercurrent with Sammy and my doubts about the summer recruits, then it was merely reflective of how we were no longer singing off the same hymn sheet. I can remember picking Vitor for a game against Chelsea once and, if I am honest, I did so to try and prove a point: to show that he wasn't at the standard we needed. Having told me to pick the new recruits, Rafa said I should have left him out for a game like that against one of the better teams around.

"If he can't play against Chelsea, what's he doing here?" I asked, reasonably enough. The irony was that we won that game 2-0 and that he actually played okay.

I was effectively speaking up for the academy then and I will continue to do so to this day. I think the criticism the set-up at Liverpool has received has been unjust. How can people say it has underperformed? Liverpool reached the FA Youth Cup final three years out of four, beating Manchester City in 2006, United in 2007 and losing to Arsenal in 2009. People say it is not about winning trophies. Okay, I accept that. But, to my mind, we did bring through players who were good enough. The only problem was that they were never subsequently given a proper opportunity to show how good they were in the first team.

The progress the likes of Martin Kelly, Jay Spearing, Jonathan Flanagan and Jack Robinson have made since proves that the academy is not a busted flush, but I think there have been others who could have been given more of a chance. But they all missed out.

I also get uptight when I hear people say Rafa brought them through – he didn't. They were already in the system when he arrived and, if anything, he could have given them a chance earlier. He may have played Jack Robinson at Hull City in what turned out to be his final game in charge at the end of the 2009/2010 season, but that was a political selection to me, one that came too late. It should never have been like that.

Flooding the place with foreign youngsters represented a scattergun approach to youth recruitment. Liverpool had a Spanish chief scout in Eduardo and so he inevitably looked to Spain a lot because that is what he knew best. The emphasis was all wrong. If the club had looked under its own nose and chosen to put their faith in more local players, things could have worked out better.

Even some of the better foreign kids that were recruited suffered from the same lack of opportunities that affected the local lads like Adam Hammill and Danny Guthrie. I understand the competition for places is fierce and intense, but I was surprised Nemeth never got more of a chance to progress into the first team. He was an out-and-out goalscorer for me, who would have come on leaps and bounds just by working with better calibre players.

And, if Liverpool wanted a footballing centre-half to bring the ball out and develop play, I thought Mikel San Jose was worth a bet. The rumour is they sold him for three million Euros to Athletic Bilbao, with an opportunity to bring him back should they need to. Whether they didn't feel he was strong enough physically to cope with the Premier League I don't know. I have also heard it suggested that Mikel was sold to raise money because of the problems at the club at the time. But to me he was good at bringing the ball out and developing play. He's not doing too badly in La Liga now, either, which says a lot about his ability.

Still, my problems were starting to pile up and it wasn't just with Rafa. Angel Vales worked alongside me, but only ever reluctantly. He really wanted to be with the first team. He was very much on top of the scientific approach that plays an increasingly important part in the game now, overseeing the number of players who were training and things like the pitch sizes required for the first team. A lot of the exercises in training these days are short and sharp. They last three minutes and then you do them again. The players train with heart monitors, which gauge how hard they are pushing themselves at certain times. All of that stuff opened my eyes to what was required at the top end of the Premier League in the modern era, and that was what Angel tended to do.

Angel had been brought in to look after the reserves and the first team, but when he was stood with me he became increasingly frustrated that he could not see what was going on with the seniors working with Rafa. He didn't want second-hand information. He wanted to see everything with his own eyes. Basically, his mind was often elsewhere.

One of the first times I realised he wasn't happy was when we went to the Dallas Cup. We turned up at Melwood the day we were due to fly out and John Wright, who was one of the kitmen then, weighed all the bags to make sure we were all within the permitted weight. I think 19kg was the maximum, and all our bags weighed 17kg or 18kg. But Angel's suitcase weighed in at 6kg, which I thought was strange because we were supposed to be away for 10 days. Then, when we got to the airport, it transpired his passport had expired. Surprise, surprise.

We also had problems with three of the Hungarian lads – Nemeth, Simon and Gulacsi – who did not have the correct visas, so they followed us across the Pond three or four days later. Rafa also made Angel come out late too, which he wasn't happy about. He clearly didn't want to be there.

I let the players go to a shopping mall for a couple of hours the day before one of the games, and he questioned whether that was the right thing to do. "But I can't keep them locked up in their rooms all day," I responded. That was genuinely how I felt, but he was still unimpressed.

Things deteriorated really from there, and continued apace once we had returned to England. In general, the last place he wanted to be

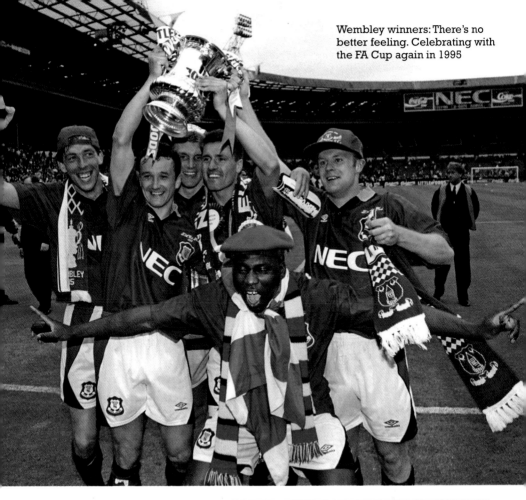

Wembley winners: There's no better feeling. Celebrating with the FA Cup again in 1995

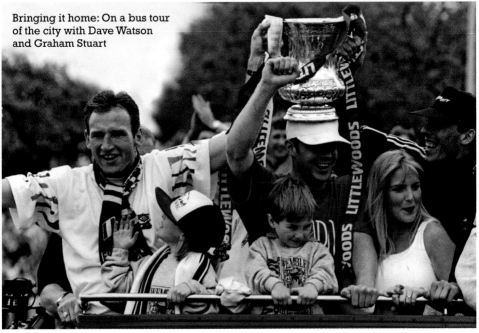

Bringing it home: On a bus tour of the city with Dave Watson and Graham Stuart

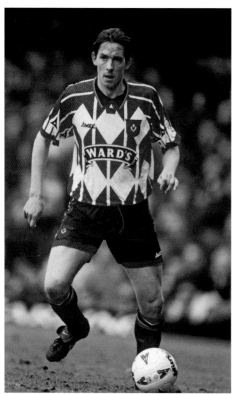

A Blade: Appearing for Sheffield United, where I teamed up with Howard Kendall again

Putting in the graft: A gym session during my stint at Blackpool in 2000, time ticking on my playing career

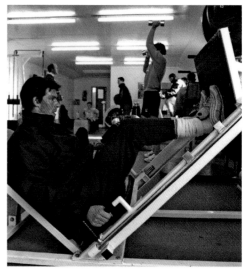

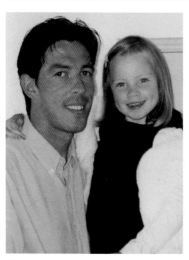

The most important job of all – being a Dad. Me and Scarlet

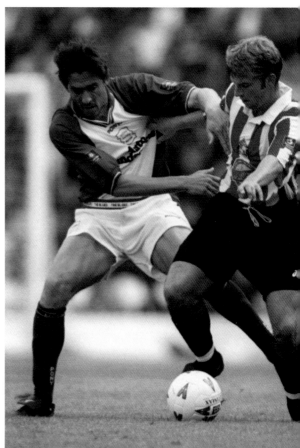

At Birmingham City, where injury scuppered my chances of a new deal

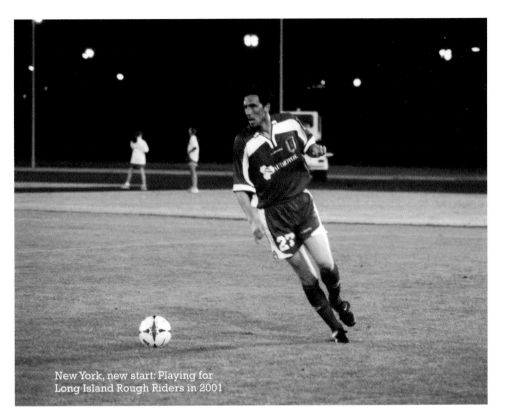

New York, new start: Playing for
Long Island Rough Riders in 2001

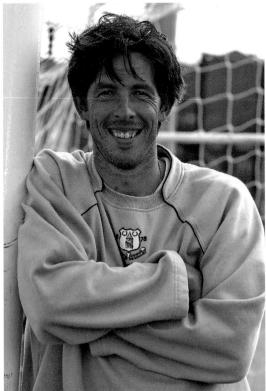

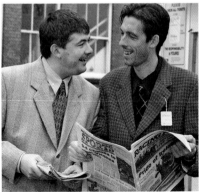

Happy days: A trip to the races with
a good mate of mine, snooker player
John Parrott and enjoying life as an
Everton coach at Finch Farm, left

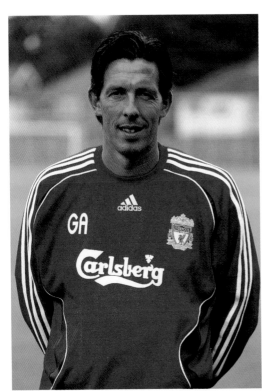

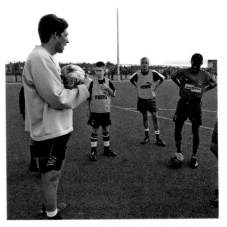

Rising stars: I loved
passing on my
experience to the
next generation

Champs again: Back at
Melwood (left) and at Anfield
with the title trophy that my
reserves team won in 2008

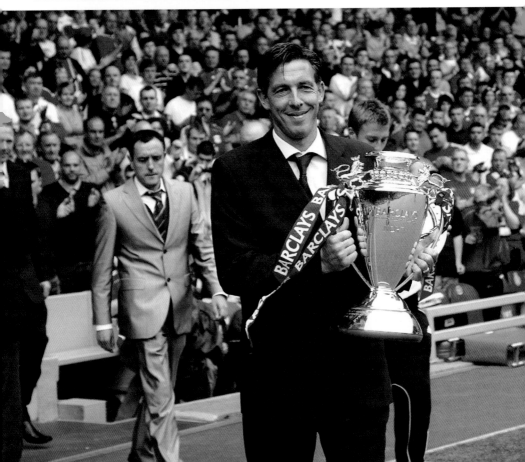

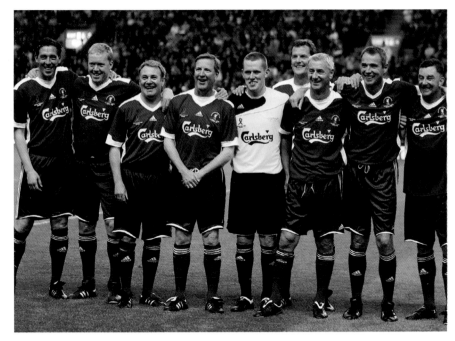

Old boys' reunion: Back with some of my former Liverpool team-mates for the Hillsborough Disaster Memorial Match at Anfield in 2009. Below, right: Deep in thought in the dugout as the manager of Stockport County – a tough job

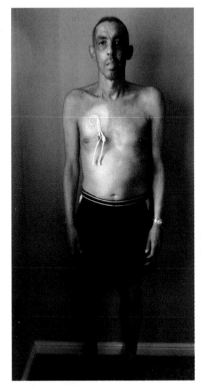

Harrowing: This picture says it all as the illness takes hold

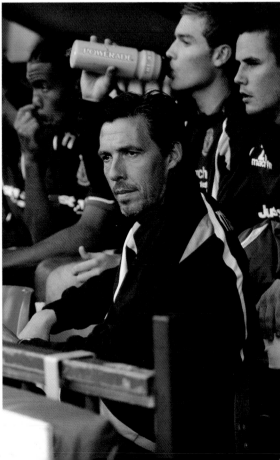

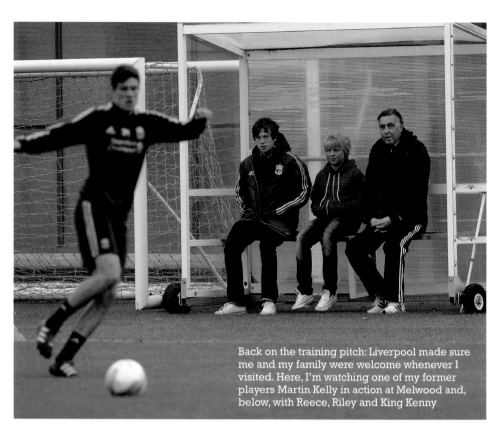

Back on the training pitch: Liverpool made sure me and my family were welcome whenever I visited. Here, I'm watching one of my former players Martin Kelly in action at Melwood and, below, with Reece, Riley and King Kenny

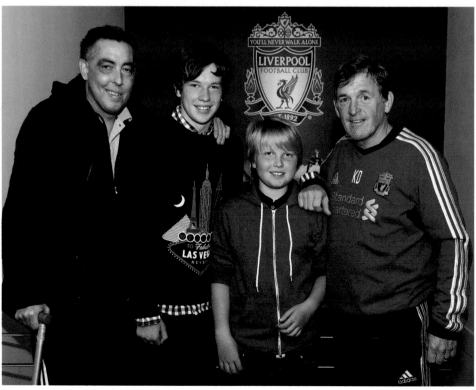

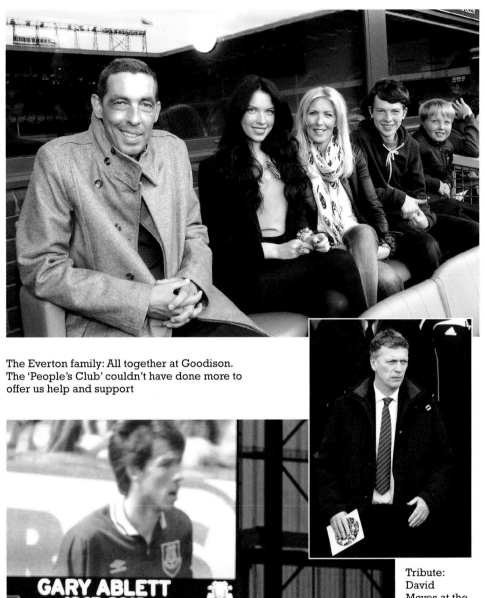

The Everton family: All together at Goodison. The 'People's Club' couldn't have done more to offer us help and support

GARY ABLETT
1965-2012

Tribute: David Moyes at the Anglican Cathedral service and a round of applause before the Blues' FA Cup third round tie against Tamworth

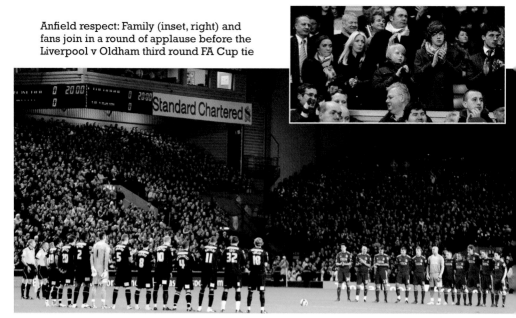

Anfield respect: Family (inset, right) and fans join in a round of applause before the Liverpool v Oldham third round FA Cup tie

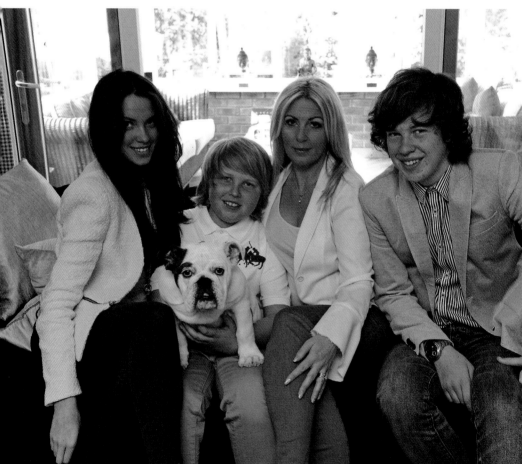

Scarlet, Riley, Jacqueline and Reece – and Bella the bulldog

was with me, but Rafa said I had to get him to coach. But I couldn't get someone to coach who wasn't interested in doing that. Angel was a serious man and he wanted to stand there with his stopwatch and blow the whistle on his timings – that's it. I felt I was being made a scapegoat for someone who didn't want to coach.

Eventually, Angel and Rafa fell out, too. Angel's disillusionment with his role was in many ways a challenge to Rafa. So a friendship that had lasted something like 20 years just ended, abruptly. Within a few weeks of Rafa being given his new contract by Tom Hicks and George Gillett in the summer of 2008, Angel was sacked. Sadly, he wasn't the only one. Lots of people left the club – and the academy especially – around that time. Good men, who had given unstinting service to Liverpool in the hope of seeing the club move on. Of course, that doesn't mean I – or anyone else – deserved a job for life. There are, however, ways of treating people, and too many of those who left weren't afforded the respect or dignity they were due.

Looking back, I think as soon as Rafa got his new deal and was effectively thrust into a position of even greater power at the club, it was the beginning of the end for anyone who had crossed him. If you weren't in his gang, you could forget it. He kept hold of people who weren't good enough, in my opinion, and I felt very much on my own, constantly trying to fight fires. The enjoyment went out of the job and we didn't have a great season on the pitch. Players like Emiliano Insua stepped up to the first team and we never had a settled side.

It just seemed that there was always an undercurrent, which was unnerving. There was too much politics about the place, and it all felt too sinister. I went to see the manager about a new contract and was told the priority was to sort out the first team, not the second string. I couldn't complain about that, but after a while I went back and asked where mine was. I was just told they hadn't got round to it yet.

Things came to a head when we returned from Holland, where we had been playing in a tournament. Upon our arrival back at Melwood, Billy Stewart, the goalkeeping coach, was sacked almost as soon as he had got off the coach. He was told that the goalkeepers weren't progressing as much as the club hoped and that there would be changes. But he didn't sign the goalkeepers. He was presented with players by the first-team hierarchy, and had to mould them as best he could.

If they could treat Billy like that then, given everything that had gone on that season, I thought it could easily be me next. The following day I was meant to be off, but said to Jacqueline that I was going into work to find out what was going on. Rafa wasn't in at first, but I was determined to get to the bottom of whether I had a future at the club so I hung around for a couple of hours and waited for him.

He eventually arrived, and there was a bit of idle chat between us: how the tournament had gone; who had played well for us. It was an uncomfortable conversation because both of us knew that wasn't really the issue at hand.

"I fancy a change," Rafa eventually said. "You'll not be working here any more."

I wasn't totally surprised, but fought my corner. "Why? What have I done wrong."

"Nothing – I just feel the time is right for a change. I have no problem with your coaching, I think you are professional and I would recommend you to people."

"So why am I going, then?"

He never gave me a plausible answer. I've heard all sorts of stories since: Sami Hyypia had been offered the reserve job as part of a new contract the club had been discussing with him. Or that John McMahon, who worked at Tranmere Rovers and who eventually replaced me, had been lined up for months. You don't know what to believe when things like that happen. Rumours are just part and parcel of life at a big club like Liverpool, after all.

But to accomplish what we had achieved and to go from being assured I was doing well when I asked about Alex Miller's job to now being bundled out of the door almost on the quiet I still find really strange. But, at the end of the day, maybe I just wasn't in the gang because I had my own ideas and my own opinions. I would speak my mind and I was never a 'yes' man.

In many respects, looking back, my coaching career at Liverpool seems to have taken a similar route to my time as a player there. I didn't conform to how everyone else wanted when I was a player in the first team and, likewise, if I didn't think a player was good enough for the reserves then I wasn't going to just pick him on the manager's say-so.

Quite probably I said too much. Maybe if I had kept my mouth shut and had done as Rafa had told me to, then I wouldn't have been sacked. I'll never know.

16

Managing

Management had always been something I had wanted to test myself at one day so, when the call came from Stockport County in the summer of 2009, there was no hesitation on my part. I jumped at it. Firstly, it was a job. Secondly, it was an opportunity to put into practice the good bits I had learned from Rafa Benitez, and the tips I had picked up from playing under the likes of Kenny Dalglish and Howard Kendall.

I knew it would not be easy. Stockport had just about survived in League One the previous season, despite winning only once in their final nine games and having slipped into administration, a process that had seen them incur a 10-point deduction. That had left them teetering a point above the cut-off in the final table. Regardless, I still really thought I could make a difference, particularly as things appeared to be looking up. Jim Melrose, the former Leicester City striker, was heading a consortium that comprised of two other men, Mark Maguire and Graham Gallagher, who said that the club would be coming out of administration at the beginning of August.

When that happened, I would sign my contract. Stockport were offering a salary of £100,000-a-year and a package that included medical bills for the family, a car, a mobile phone and expenses. It was an attractive offer, and one that was too good to turn down, but that just fuelled my enthusiasm for the task I was taking on. I had big plans for the future of Stockport County.

The squad had lots of shortcomings and limitations, clearly, but I had been promised we would be out of administration shortly and then I would be able to put more of my own stamp on things. I would be able to bring in my own players and reshape the playing squad, and make County my team. Until then, it was a case of making the best of what we had. That wasn't too much of a hardship because, in six weeks, we'd have new, permanent owners and we could move forward.

Jim organised a pre-season barbecue for the staff and the playing squad at the training ground, Manor Farm, and we had a great time. The lads ordered me up to sing on the karaoke – 'You'll Never Walk Alone' had been picked for me, inevitably – and I belted that out before handing the microphone on.

My staff included Steve Jones, who had been recommended to me by Mick McDermott, whom I had played with at Long Island Rough Riders, and he was a fitness coach. Steve had never met the players prior to that get-together, had never even been in a room with them before, and so when they selected a Britney Spears track for him to sing, it could have gone two ways. It is to his credit that he had everyone in hysterics, and that served to break the ice with the squad. They immediately thought: 'He'll do for us. He's one of us.'

If we were going to get anywhere, I knew team spirit would be vital. I wanted us to play football the right way, the way I had been schooled by Ronnie Moran and Roy Evans on the pitches at Melwood. Pass and move, pass and move. Keep it simple. But if there was no camaraderie within the squad, we'd get nowhere.

Hughie McAuley came on board to help me. John Ward was my assistant to begin with, but Aidy Boothroyd offered him a job at Colchester United and, understandably, John decided to take it. So I turned to Hughie, someone who I could trust implicitly. Someone who had helped me out unbelievably when I was first at Liverpool, and someone who wouldn't blow smoke up my arse if he didn't think I was doing the right things. It is easy when you are manager for everyone just to say: "Yes boss, you're right boss, of course boss, you're the best boss, it's their fault boss." I knew Hughie would be straight with me if I stepped out of line.

I quickly settled into my new routine. I would set off from Tarleton at 7.30am for the training ground, have a cup of tea and a slice of toast with my staff when I got there, and find out who was injured and who would be available on the Saturday. But, driving over to Stockport in the build up to our opening game of the season, away at Oldham Athletic, it felt different. My mind was racing. Who to pick? What formation to play?

There was more pressure on me than I had experienced before because the results were more important for Stockport, and more important for the players and the fans. I wanted to win when I was in charge of the reserves for Liverpool, but really that was as much about bringing players through. Winning was the be all and end all for me now, like it had been when I was a player at Liverpool – only now I was the one in the firing line.

We drew that opening game at Boundary Park, and the goalless draw felt like a satisfying start for me. A clean sheet was important and, climbing on board the team bus home afterwards, there was a real sense that we had achieved something. It was a start. We were off the mark and up and running. Even when we subsequently lost at Huddersfield Town in the Carling Cup, and twice more at Edgeley Park in the league to Bristol Rovers and Carlisle United, I didn't get too down-beat, and my first win as a League One manager arrived on August 22, 2009.

We had travelled down to Brighton the night before and put on what turned out to be one of our best performances of the season, winning 4-2 in a real roller-coaster of a game. Brighton took the lead before Carl Baker equalised, and then he put us ahead in the opening 10 minutes of the second half. We conceded again within a few minutes before Brighton had two players sent off, and found themselves down to nine. Carl completed a brilliant hat-trick from the penalty spot following the second red card before our own Liam Bridcutt was sent off six minutes from time. It felt like sheer agony on the touchline as the clock ticked down.

I wished I was out there trying to influence things instead of relaying instructions frantically from the sidelines, but thankfully Oli Johnson scored with a minute of normal time left to thrust us further clear. The final whistle brought the sort of rush I'd felt at Wembley with Liverpool, or even when Everton had achieved their great escape against Wimbledon. There is an overwhelming sense of pride, that what you have worked on all week on the training ground has come together.

Carl was first-class that day, and I knew he was too good for us. He moved to Coventry City in the New Year for £175,000, and I'm still in touch with him. Not so much because I was his manager for six months, but because what I have gone through since, Carl and his family can also relate to. One of the hardest things I had to do during my time at Stockport was to tell Carl his brother had died from leukaemia. Carl's family were trying to get hold of him to tell him but without success, so they eventually phoned the club. We were out on the training pitch and the physio came out to tell me. It became my responsibility to inform Carl and, in those circumstances, there is no way of making bad news sound good.

He was in bits. I sent him home immediately and told him to get back in touch when he was ready. No rush. No pressure. Just when he was ready. We were due to play at Yeovil Town that weekend but, on the Thursday before our trip down south, my mobile phone rang. It was Carl saying he wanted to play. We picked him up en route and he showed incredible bravery that day, netting twice in a 2-2 draw. Each time he scored, he lifted his shirt up to reveal a message in memory of his brother that was on his T-shirt.

A week later we were at home to Leyton Orient and I met Carl's mum before the match. She asked me to thank all of the team for rallying round behind Carl on her behalf. "Why don't you say that to them?" I asked. So she came into the dressing room and virtually gave the pre-match team-talk for me, telling everyone what a great club Stockport was and, if we stuck together, we'd be okay. I hardly had to say anything. We won 2-1 with a late goal from Greg Tansey. What had been an emotional day for everyone had finished in the perfect way.

Off the pitch, though, I was beginning to become alarmed by the lack of progress being made by Jim's consortium in buying the club. We beat Leyton Orient on 19 September, but were firmly in the grip of administration with no sign of a resolution. What had happened to being under new ownership and looking to progress by August?

Jim had been that confident of taking over that he had a string of people coming up to the club to work, who shouldn't have been there. Andy May, who used to be at Manchester City, worked alongside Craig Madden and helped out with the youth team. I thought he was a full-time member of staff, but it was only a few weeks later that I realised Jim had given him the job to be confirmed when he formally took over the club. As it was, the administrators belatedly realised what was happening and stepped in, saying that wasn't on. But, as a result, Jim started to take a back seat and the regular phone calls to me stopped. I haven't spoken to him for God knows how long now.

Although the administrators were in charge, Mark Maguire effectively ran the club from my point of view, and he did quite well in my opinion. But that wasn't the point. I had been promised all these things – money, ambition, an opportunity to get the club progressing – but nothing ever materialised. And so the problems snowballed.

I had wanted to give our Manor Farm training ground a complete overhaul and make it somewhere the players would enjoy spending time. The 'to do' list was lengthy. I wanted to improve the changing rooms and shower facilities. The physio room, which I hoped to switch to the area being used as a gym, would become a classroom with the gym instead taking up two-thirds of what was, back then, the canteen. Ah, the canteen. The oven needed a new grill and a new oven door. This wasn't quite up to the standards of 'Masterchef'. Not yet, anyway.

Some students from the local college came in and did some painting to spruce the buildings up, but trying to put the rest of my plans into practice was like banging my head against a brick wall.

Take the gym, for example. We were paying hundreds of pounds a month on rental for equipment, most of which did not work. Steve Jones tried to fix a deal with someone to get rid of it all and bring some new equipment in, but the administrators wouldn't let us. It was a false economy, but they just refused to budge.

Then there was the Edgeley Park pitch. We shared it with Sale Sharks rugby union side and, because of the amount of use it had, it resembled a beach. The day I was offered the coaching job at Ipswich Town, I was doing my FA Pro Licence with Gus Poyet. He had photos on his phone of the pitch from the 2009/10 season when Brighton played us and was showing everyone on the course how bad it was. That pitch was a hindrance to us. It affected how we played. I'd wanted us to play a passing game because it was what I believed in, but really we couldn't have played like that on that surface. There was no chance.

We needed to add to the squad, too. As a team we weren't old enough, strong enough, or physical enough, mentally and emotionally. We would become disheartened at the first sign of a setback. One of the restrictions of having administrators in place was that we were only ever allowed to have a squad of 20 players. Yet, when I took over, half of the lads hadn't been anywhere near the first team and we were using 17 and 18-year-olds who would tell you they were ready to play but, in truth, they weren't.

Look at the players the club had sold in recent seasons. Liam Dickinson moved to Derby for £750,000. Then there was Anthony Pilkington, who moved on to Huddersfield Town and eventually into the Premier League with Norwich City. There was also Tommy Rowe, James Tunnicliffe and Jermaine Easter. If Stockport had managed to keep them all together, they would have had some side. I'd look at the opposition team sheet every week and someone would say to me, matter-of-factly: "Oh, he used to be here."

I had to wheel and deal, offloading players on loan to Conference sides usually and trying to bring others in on short-term, temporary deals. We ended up using 33 players that season. The team was never settled. The turnover in playing staff was huge. Results dipped, and everything then becomes a vicious circle. From October 17, 2009 to January 19, 2010 we did not win a single league game. Actually, worse still, we did not win a single league point.

I wasn't overly hard on the players because they were struggling to cope with everything that was going on anyway. Form had drained away, confidence was shattered, and I just felt that if I had come down on them hard that it wouldn't have helped matters. It wouldn't have provoked a positive reaction. Don't get me wrong: there were times when I would shake them up after a game, but it got to the stage where I just felt that I was repeating the same things to the players and nothing was sinking in. I don't think they were mature enough to handle what was going on.

The fact that we were a club still in administration, despite all the promises, created an environment which offered the players an excuse. But the reality was we didn't have it as bad as other teams who have experienced administration. We could still go away the night before games. That was never in doubt. Yes, there was a budget in terms of what we could eat, but it wasn't a problem and we still managed to eat healthily. If you compare what Peter Reid went through at Plymouth Argyle, with players not being paid and a constant worry over whether the club would suddenly cease to exist, then my lot were on easy street in contrast. Plymouth had it so much worse. Their wages kept being deferred, but we got paid on time every month.

What I would say is that, on the Pro-Licence coaching course, there should be a section that deals with what you do if your club goes into administration. It is happening more and more these days and, if your club does find itself in the mire, then it is difficult to cope with. Some of the players would come to me in the week and say: "Gaffer, I don't know where my head is." They'd tell me about how they would jump in the car after games and the next minute they'd be home, but they wouldn't be able to remember anything about the journey because their minds had been racing. The uncertainty was getting to them all, and that was pretty scary really.

Some of them cared. It was just too tough for the majority of the players. Even some of the senior ones, who I'd always envisaged would be there for the club throughout, went missing at the end of the season. Injury this, injury that...that all disappointed me on a personal level, but it goes to show the frame of mind they were in because, as the results disintegrated around us, there was no hiding place.

We brought a psychologist in called Alistair Smith, who worked with the lads individually and as a group. He worked for nothing, but even he struggled to fathom some of them out. The environment may have been poor but, overall, I think the players lacked responsibility. And you can add to that humility and integrity.

Steve Jones' partner, Jeanette, was a dietician and she tried to help them, telling them what the right things to eat were. But her advice was ignored. Jeanette and Jacqueline had both been to a game at Norwich and we all stopped off at a service station on the way home. The players went straight to KFC, stocking up on Popcorn chicken and the like. Jeanette was pulling her hair out.

That showed the immaturity of the players. I used to tell them to act now, take charge of their futures and make the most of what they had now. "Don't wait," I'd say. "You've not got as much time on your side as you think." But too many were happy to accept second best. They blamed others, instead of looking at themselves.

It is amazing the amount of resistance Steve met when he tried to get the players in the gym, for example. Amazing because now everyone has gone their separate ways, those same lads will ring Steve up asking him to sort a fitness programme out for them. They are the same programmes he wanted to implement three years ago.

Early in the New Year we managed to bring in five players. David Perkins arrived on loan from Colchester United and he did really well for us. Danny Swailes and Richie Partridge came from MK Dons, and then there were Jabo Ibehre and Jemal Johnson, who also came in from the same club. They shared a house, which probably wasn't the best idea. Jabo was just a quiet lad. Let's just say Jemal wasn't – he was a headache. There were complaints about noise coming from the apartment. They soon fell out. I spoke to Paul Ince and Carl Robinson about the situation, but it was on my watch and my problem. I just felt he needed to respect himself a bit more. He'd been on the phone at the wrong times and then, when you needed to get hold of him, he wouldn't answer. We tried to bring disciplinary action against him, but he was the one who was protected, not the club.

It wasn't just the players who were suffering. As the season wore on,

I became increasingly self-reflective as well. Could I have done better? Should I have done more? What had I done well? Should I have been more pragmatic and altered our style of play? Looking back, I know now that I hadn't really appreciated what I was letting myself in for by going to Stockport because I genuinely thought the club would be out of administration sooner rather than later. That feels naïve now. Having said that, I probably still would have taken the job, even if I had been told back there and then in the summer that there was no timescale for how long the club would be in the hands of the administrators. I just would not have harboured the same aspirations over what I might have been able to achieve in the short or long-term.

In hindsight, I am sure I could have done things better. Maybe I should have been more open to change over my desire to play the game properly when the state of our pitch was not conducive to that. But this was my first managerial job. My first opportunity to do things my way. Perhaps that sense of ambition clouded my judgement.

There were times throughout the season where I wondered what might have been. I had been offered a job to go to the United Arab Emirates to coach Al Ain's Under-19s. Mick McDermott, whom I had played with for Long Island Rough Riders, was a fitness and conditioning coach there and said there was an opportunity to join him. I had received an offer after leaving Liverpool and I spoke with them but, almost at the same time, Stockport got in touch.

Being truthful, the kids didn't want to go to Dubai. They had their own lives here and it would have been hard to up sticks and move somewhere we had never been before. But, when we did eventually go for a holiday over there, they actually loved it. "Dad, we should have come here." They absolutely loved it.

It wasn't all bad that season, of course. There were some (relatively) good times as well, and I have to say that the Stockport County supporters were very patient and positive throughout what must have felt a depressingly difficult season. I couldn't reward them as much as I wanted to, but I remember the reaction to a 0-0 draw at Carlisle United in January, which ended a run of 12 straight league defeats.

We celebrated in the changing room that night as though we had won the league itself. The lads were so used to coming off the pitch having got a good beating that there was just a huge sense of relief for them. We'd got a point. Just one point, but it was massive for them. It was huge for the staff and the supporters who had travelled north. Afterwards, it felt like we had pulled off some giant-killing act in the FA Cup, beating a Manchester United or a Chelsea. The whole atmosphere in the changing room changed in an instant because of the result, and we came away thinking that this could be the turning point. As it was, while we drew at home to Brighton in the next game, we then lost away at Southampton and the rot duly set in again.

I always tried to approach each game positively and I never ever thought we would get smashed. But it always threatened to wear you down. At the start of the season, Saturday afternoon was always something to look forward to. Yet, when you can't buy a result, you need a good family behind you and people you can trust alongside you to get you through it all. I was lucky enough to have that, and I would always going into training on a Monday morning aiming to try and put things right again following a defeat at the weekend. I always regarded the next game as the one in which our fortunes would turn.

If you were to ask a lot of the managers we came up against, they always felt we would give them a game to a certain point. While it was 0-0 and while it was a game of football then, in my opinion, we were as good as anyone in the league. When we got it down and passed it, we were fine. But, once we had conceded one or two goals, we would simply collapse. If someone wanted to batter us and rough us up, then we couldn't stand up to that. We were too young, we weren't physical enough. We were basically powerless to stop it. And so, by the end of the season, Saturday had become the day you dreaded most of all. I knew where the players were mentally at that point, and they were not capable of turning things around.

We had all known it was coming, but we were finally relegated from League One in early April following a 3-1 home defeat to Yeovil Town. The dressing room was like a morgue afterwards, but there weren't tears or anything like that. We had done badly for so long that everyone had got used to the idea of dropping out of the division. It had felt inevitable for a while. I wouldn't say it was a relief to have our fate confirmed but, in my own mind, what had occurred and the manner in which it had all happened crystallised what had to come next.

I wasn't planning on giving up, though. I started jotting some notes down in a diary, things we needed to do now to give us a chance of coming straight back up the following season. We needed bigger players, lads who were physically and mentally stronger, more athletic, players who had better stamina and were more explosive. We needed to find a balance between youth and experience. We needed leaders in the side – and characters.

If I am being brutally honest, of the 20 players we had on the books at the end of that 2009/10 season, I was planning to give maybe four or five of them another year's contract. The rest could go. It would have meant a tough, tough summer in terms of recruitment and rebuilding, but that is where the club was at. It needed a complete and total revamp. My first season as a manager had been a nightmare in terms of the results we'd achieved, but my enthusiasm hadn't dipped. I still had my plans and my goals. I still had my dreams. At the start of pre-season training, I would lay down the law to everyone and we would start afresh in League Two.

* * * * * * * * * * * * * * *

On April 20, 2010, Stockport County's administrators accepted a bid of exclusivity from the self-styled '2015 Consortium', a new group of businessmen who had emerged from the ether and were interested in buying the club. Jim Melrose was still in the background – somewhere – but his own bid had effectively lapsed. I knew this would have implications for me. The new prospective owners had no loyalty towards me, and the club they were trying to buy had just been relegated. Worry began to set in.

A number of people in the consortium also knew Jim Gannon, the former Stockport manager, and rumours soon started swirling that he would be coming back and taking over in time for the following season. It was a difficult period, exacerbated by the fact that no one picked up the phone to shed any light on whether we would be part of the club's future or not. That's football I suppose. Things change overnight. Loyalty is the first thing to go out of the window.

In that situation, you have to look after number one. I told my staff that, if a job was available elsewhere, they should think seriously about taking it. We might not be here for two weeks, let alone two years.

Hughie had received an offer to work at the academy at Perth Glory, where Robbie Fowler was playing at the time. But he just felt that, at his age, it was too far for him to go. He'd miss his grandkids too much being on the other side of the world, so he stuck around. Paul Gerrard, my goalkeeping coach whom people will know from his time at Everton, was another I told to scout around for opportunities. Paul was good at his job and like everyone else, he deserved some sort of security. As for me, I'd received some phone calls from members of the youth set-up at Everton saying that they'd heard I was going back to Liverpool. Rafa looked to be on his way out after a difficult season in which the early exit from the Champions League had constituted a massive blow, and the club failed to finish in the top four as well. I suppose part of me was thinking he was getting a taste of his own medicine, but I didn't revel in his misfortune. I spoke to a few people but, like most rumours, the speculation came to nothing and there would be no emotional homecoming this time.

I would have gone, definitely. At first it might have been difficult no longer being the boss and no longer having the final say on things, but I'm sure I would have adapted pretty quickly. It was Liverpool after all. Instead, I carried on, although it became increasingly obvious to me that the sack was coming.

For the final few weeks of that season, we were completely in the dark as to what was happening behind the scenes. No one communicated with us. I tried to get in touch with the consortium to find out their plans, but the administrators wouldn't ring up and pass on their numbers to me. My reign as Stockport manager was ending in the same fashion as most of it had been run: with me banging my head against a brick wall, seeking answers and getting fobbed off.

The trouble was that, for Stockport's sake, decisions had to be made now. They couldn't afford to go into the new season, in League Two, playing catch up in terms of their pre-season preparations and scrambling around for players. There was so much work to be done and it needed to be done in April not July, when everyone reported back. The wheels had to be put in motion, the rebuilding work commenced with a view to recovering the following season.

It is my understanding that part of the problem was that the 2015 Consortium didn't think I should be their concern. They wanted to wash their hands of me and my staff and move on, but the terms of employment we were working under meant it wasn't as straight forward as that. One day I received a call from the administrators asking if I could get all the staff to attend a meeting at the training ground. Presumably, it was to tell everyone that our services were no longer required, but an hour before the meeting was due to take place it was mysteriously cancelled. That was par for the course. We all feared what was likely to happen, but no one ever communicated with us effectively and we ended up lurching along in this horrendous state of limbo.

I was in contact with the League Managers' Association constantly towards the end – Graham Mackrell was my point of reference – and they helped me enormously, fighting for my rights. When the end came, ironically enough, I was actually in Dubai on holiday with Jacqueline and the kids. It was hardly a surprise, but it put a bit of a downer on the trip. Graham called to say I was getting the sack. In total, I got £11,000 in compensation.

There wasn't too much time to feel sorry for myself as Al Ain came calling again and, this time, we were all keen to give it a go in Dubai, the kids included. It represented a clean break from England, a new start and the job on offer – assistant-coach of the first team – was a good one. The coach had been promoted from the Under-17s and had been told that if he didn't get help in, they would struggle.

I was offered 120,000 Euros tax free, accommodation, a car, regular flights home, and I was negotiating to try and get the cost of schooling for the kids added onto the package. Everything was put in front of the Sheikh. We waited anxiously for a decision, all of us willing him to say yes. But, in the end, he didn't want to go English with his coaching staff after all. He went Brazilian instead. We had lost out again.

* * * * * * * * * * * * * * * *

I'd had my fingers burned at Stockport but, if I am honest, I would still want all that hassle now. It was disappointing the way it had all turned out, but I know I went into the job with the best of intentions. Football isn't fair, I know that. I learnt that at a young age, but my fledgling experiences as a young manager were a great education in so many ways, a good learning curve. It certainly opened my eyes to the world of management.

As for putting me off, no chance. I think I have so much more to offer. I want my teams to play the right way. We were doing things the right way, but we just didn't have the personnel on the playing side who could handle want we wanted. During the last 16 months, I've thought about a return to management a lot. The question is just whether or not I could do it now. Whether I could cope every day out on the field, or whether I'd have to let someone else do all that for me.

That's not really me, though. I would want to be involved, I'd want to be at the coal face, working with the players, enjoying the banter. Not tucked away inside, or overviewing everyone else. That is the dilemma I have and that is where having cancer makes its mark in other ways. Right now I don't know whether my body will let me do that again, and I don't know if it ever will.

It has been suggested to me that the stress of management possibly contributed to my illness. The doctors have said stress isn't good. But I have to say I didn't feel particularly stressed at the time. Yes, we were losing, but I genuinely enjoyed going into work. I liked the hassle. Maybe I bottled it up. Maybe I was suffering from pressure, I'll never know. Making sure I am healthy again is my first priority, but there's nothing more I'd like than to be on the touchline on a Saturday afternoon again, seeing the team I've worked with all week, the players I've pinned my faith in, giving their all.

17

Full Circle

"Alright, Giblet."

Since breaking into the Liverpool team all those years ago, Kenny has always called me that. Not 'Abbo,' or anything, just 'Giblet.' I've no idea why, and he probably couldn't tell you himself. But when I walked into Melwood in the late autumn of 2011 to find Kenny standing there in reception with a beaming smile plastered across his face, that familiar greeting transported me back to my playing days and into the dressing room at Anfield.

Things had come full circle for me: back at Liverpool, Kenny back as manager, me back hanging onto The King's every word. Only this time we weren't talking about marking the opposition right winger.

There had always been an open invitation to myself and the boys to pop down to the training ground since Kenny took over the reins again and, finally, I took him up on the offer in half-term in October 2011. Reece and Riley came and we had a brilliant day. I'd always get a fair few texts off Kenny, but it was great to speak to him face to face and chat about things. He asked about the family and how everyone was and, of course, with his wife Marina's own battle against breast cancer he appreciates my situation and what I am going through. But, as with David Moyes when he came to visit me in hospital that first time, the talk soon turned to football.

Needless to say, Kenny was enjoying being back at Liverpool. It's home for him and the positivity he radiates is there for everyone to see. Sure, to everyone else, Liverpool is not the same club as when Kenny left, but to Kenny it is still the best in the world. And, as such, you won't hear him talking the opposition up or anything like that.

I've seen a lot of his press conferences on Sky or the LFC TV channel because I'm in the house a lot, and I love it when he says things like: "Yes, they've got good players, but I'm sure they'll be worried about us as well." It just plants that little seed of doubt in the opposition. That Liverpool won't be pushovers under Kenny Dalglish. That he'll defend the club to the end. What more, as a Liverpool supporter or player, could you wish for?

Kenny put his reputation on the line to an extent by returning to the club, although he does not see it like that. He just believes he is trying to help Liverpool out and that they have actually done him the favour by bringing him back. It won't be easy for him to win titles and cups again because football has changed so much from when Liverpool were top dogs in terms of money and stadia. But the principles Kenny cherishes still hold true today. If you pass the ball and move better than your opponents, you'll win more games than you lose. It's simple, really, and you can see that starting to take hold now in the performances.

In addition, I detect that he's re-instilled into the club what Liverpool is all about. The club had grown cold in my opinion, detached almost, but there is a warmth to it again now and that is down to Kenny. He treats everyone the same and he wants everyone to be the best they can be – and that extends to their attitude towards people.

Although I had never really overlapped with the first team during my time as reserve coach, I know a lot of the lads. Pepe Reina came over when the boys and I were in the canteen having some tea and toast and I was talking to him about his autobiography, which was published last year. Craig Bellamy had a word with us and it was clear that he was enjoying himself this time around, more than he ever did under Rafa. "It's nice to feel wanted," he said.

Training was split into two groups: finishing and defending. Typically, Kenny ambled over to the strikers, but Reece, Riley and me took a seat in one of the portable dug-outs and watched Steve Clarke, Kenny's assistant, putting the defenders through a session. I've seen Steve and first-team coach Kevin Keen put on a session before and they're top class. Liverpool are in safe hands with those guys on the coaching staff.

It was just nice to see a few old, friendly faces again. Jamie Carragher had been up to the house with Mike Dickinson from Everton, who actually used to be his school teacher, back when Roy Hodgson was still in charge of Liverpool. I like Carra a lot. He reminds me of Roy Keane in that he speaks his mind and he believes in his opinions. More often than not, what he says is right as well.

Carra had invited me down to Melwood during one international break and I took Reece with me. I remember walking in and going up to the canteen, and you'd have thought I was a stranger rather than someone who had spent over three seasons there. "It doesn't take long to forget me, does it?" I said to Carol Farrell and Caroline Guest, the women who keep all the players happy by preparing their breakfasts and lunches.

Of course, I was teasing. The way I look has changed so much that it took a while for them to recognise me. I could see them looking, half recognising me, but not wanting to say anything in case they were wrong. That is where cancer makes other people feel awkward. I'm used to it, but when you meet up with people you haven't seen for ages it can be much more of a shock to them. When they realised who it was, they burst into tears. I seem to have that effect on people! "It's not been the same since you left," they said before proceeding to make a right fuss of me and Reece. Toast, cups of tea, you name it. Nothing was too much trouble.

It was after breakfast that I went out to watch training and, as I say, to view the session Steve and Kevin were putting on. It was fantastic. There were only six lads taking part because Melwood becomes a ghost town during international windows, but the tempo was great and the quality of the coaching was excellent. Maybe it's the coach and manager in me, but I pinched a piece of paper, grabbed a pen and started scribbling notes on what Steve and Kevin had the players doing. Hopefully, the little tips and techniques I picked up will come in handy when I am back on the touchline, putting a team of my own through their paces.

Liverpool has changed dramatically since I was there, but I still speak to some of the medical staff: people like Rob Pryce, Chris Morgan and Paul Small, all of them good lads who are very good at their jobs. Due to our friendship, Chris did the Manchester 10k run last year and raised £22,000 for The Christie. That was a tremendous sum and, hopefully, it will get used in the correct manner. Initially, he was hoping to raise only about £5,000 but, within a couple of weeks, his sponsorship had gone way beyond that and the final total was superb. I can't thank him enough for his efforts.

We were at Melwood for around three hours that day in October and, before we left, Kenny signed some books for the kids and made us promise we'd visit again. "Anytime you want to come down, just call," Kenny said. "Don't leave it long." He's a good man. A proper man with proper values, but I've come to realise, with the support I've received during this illness, that I know a lot of people like that.

Reece and Riley don't get awestruck when they're in the company of The King. It's second nature to them. It's been my life and so it has been their life, too. It's Liverpool or no one for Reece but, where Riley once used to support every team and no team, now he has certainly embraced Everton. I think it is largely down to how Everton have treated me and the lengths they go to in making sure I am okay. Ray Hall and Neil Dewsnip, good people from the academy, are in contact a lot and Mike Dickinson visits regularly. I think Riley recognises this and it's nice that he thinks he'll repay the loyalty Everton have shown his dad by supporting them.

There's also the fact that he gets spoilt rotten whenever we go to Finch Farm to factor in as well, of course! Drinks, toast, chocolate, whatever he wants... it's never far away when we're up in the coaches' office on a Saturday morning waiting for the Under-18s to start. Or, sometimes, Everton let us sit on the balcony outside David Moyes' office, which has a spectacular view of all the main pitches at Finch Farm, so we can watch the likes of Tim Cahill, Phil Neville, Phil Jagielka and the rest of the first team out in training.

Then we'll go inside and have some lunch. Usually it's me, Reece, Riley and Mike Dickinson having a bite to eat. Then Duncan Ferguson will pull up a chair and start nattering away. Riley always nods back and laughs, but he has since said to Jacqueline that he can never understand what Duncan is saying.

Ray Hall comes and sits down. So does Kevin O'Brien, one of the coaches, and before you know it there are seven or eight of us all talking away, chatting about Everton. All very matter of fact. All very natural. They make you feel so welcome and it's a great release for me and the kids. Sometimes I need that. A little reminder of life at a football club, something I perhaps took for granted before the illness set in.

* * * * * * * * * * * * * * * * *

You've already heard a bit about what Roy Keane has done for me since I've been ill. I know well enough the image Roy has from the outside. He's seen as being abrasive, confrontational. He's even considered to be trouble. To me, he is none of those things. Yes, he speaks his mind. He has strong views on a variety of subjects. But, to me, Roy has been caring, incredibly supportive and a true friend. The only time you could say he has been trouble is when he has smuggled a bag of sugary sweets onto the ward at The Christie when I was in for 12 days having treatment for my Diabetes.

I spent a week on a course with Roy doing my Pro-Licence at Warwick. We didn't particularly know each other, but we hit it off immediately. Maybe there was a connection because we had played for clubs in the north-west, at clubs who are used to winning major honours. We didn't spend that week in each other's pockets or anything, but I found that when he got up to speak during the course he had a lot of interesting views and points to make. Beyond that, though, what he said always made a lot of sense.

We kept in touch and that helped me to get the job at Ipswich Town with him, but the professional relationship we had as manager and coach does not explain just how much time he has spent with me over the past couple of years. The phone will go and it will be Roy. "I'm popping round," he'll say. But it's hardly 'popping round'. He lives in Cheshire and I'm up living near Preston. "What do you need? Papers? A magazine? Puzzle book?"

And he comes to the house, or the hospital, and we'll sit and talk about everything and anything. I really could sit and listen to Roy all day – sometimes you have to, in fairness, because he doesn't give you a chance to get a word in edgeways – but he is a smashing fella who has done so much for me.

There is obviously the story of when he brought the whole Ipswich team to see me in Addenbrooke's after they'd played up at Middlesbrough earlier in the day, but there are plenty of others. Little things to him, but gestures that mean a lot to my family and I.

When I was in The Christie last being treated for Diabetes, he told me to ask the nurse if I could pop round to his house one evening for a meal. Just to get out of the ward, to enjoy a change of scenery. I wasn't allowed to go, unfortunately, because I would have enjoyed that, but every day I was in the hospital he came to visit. Without fail. He didn't need to do that, but I'm glad he did.

Not all of the nurses shared my enthusiasm. Normally I would meet Roy in the relatives' room to keep him out of the way, but this one time he came on to the ward. It was mayhem. I actually felt bad for Roy for putting him in that position. The news soon spread that 'Keano' was in the building and there were nurses coming up from downstairs and everywhere looking for autographs, and other people, who had no real need to be there at that time, started poking their head around corners. Any excuse to see their hero.

"Everything okay?" they'd ask of me.

"Fine thanks."

"Good stuff... Oh, hi Roy, I didn't see you there. You couldn't sign this for me please, could you?"

On occasions, it was like being at the match again, with people milling around everywhere. One of the head nurses, Jackie, who was actually working on the ward, wasn't happy at all the disruption and was ready to make a complaint. I understood. She was just trying to do her job, and the place was ridiculously cluttered up. In the end, the crowds dispersed and we were left alone. I couldn't take issue with Jackie, though. She's been brilliant with me. She actually used to let me practise drawing blood out of her fingers so that, when I came home to continue my Diabetes treatment, I would know what to do.

I have two 'pens' which I inject into the stomach and, basically, I take blood level readings first thing in the morning before I eat and then I take a level before lunch, dinner and before I go to bed. It takes a bit of getting used to, but in the end you just get on with it. It's the only way.

Jackie was mad with me that day but, as for Roy, he just takes all the attention in his stride. Watching him happily signing autograph after autograph reminded me of the power footballers have these days, especially ones as good as Roy. At times, I can hear the other lads in the neighbouring beds, nudging each other and looking towards me and asking whether I really used to play. They'll know the name, but they won't particularly know the face given how puffy it has become with all the medication.

If they want to know about my career – of playing for Kenny Dalglish and clashing with Graeme Souness, or of winning the FA Cup against Manchester United at Wembley – I will tell them happily. But, if they don't, I won't go around saying I used to do this or that. I've never been like that, seeking to blow my own trumpet. If people are interested, I'll tell them. If not, I won't.

If I have learned anything from Roy over the months that have gone by, then it is that he is a massive loss to football. He's getting itchy feet since leaving Ipswich, and he wants to go back into management as soon as possible. If you are a football chairman you seriously have to ask yourself why you wouldn't want Roy Keane running your football club? Sure, he has strong views and knows just how he wants things to be done. But what's wrong with that? Surely it's better to have that than a manager who can't make up his mind? But the bottom line is that Roy Keane is a winner and, which chairman out there does not want their manager to be a winner?

A good friend does not have to be someone who is necessarily there for you every single day. It can be someone who you can ring up after two or three weeks when you haven't spoken, and just enjoy a catch up. Sometimes, it can be even longer. Given everything that has happened to me, I can still consider myself fortunate to have so many people in my life who care for me. Not just people everyone will have heard of like John Parrott, Joe Royle, Duncan Ferguson, Kenny, Jim Beglin, Alan Hansen, Jamie Carragher, Hughie McAuley, Craig Madden from Stockport, Mike Newell... the list goes on. But friends like John and Vicky Fairbrother, who'll just call one morning and invite me and Jacqueline round for a bacon butty and a cup of tea. Or Andy and Kay Gibbons, who we became friendly with when we first moved to Tarleton and who'll take us out for a meal and will only ever be a phone call away.

It is nice to know that Jacqueline and I mean something to all these people and, believe me, it does help. They're a wonderful distraction, and people whose company I enjoy. I seldom go 15 or 20 minutes without the phone going or a text buzzing through on my mobile asking how I am. When you sit back and think about that, it soon snaps you out of the low times I invariably still have.

Tarleton is a quiet village. Nothing too much goes on there, so I suppose the arrival of a host of famous faces at my front door can prompt a few double takes every now and again. This isn't me bragging. From the moment I walked into the first-team dressing room at Liverpool as a shy apprentice, mop and bucket in hand, it's all I have known and I have been lucky enough to make a lot of good friends.

I've been pals with John Parrott for years. ITV once tried to launch a rival programme to 'A Question of Sport' and wanted John to be the captain. They asked me to go and be a guest on the pilot programme and, because we lived quite close together, the car the television company sent collected us both.

We clicked, and have stayed close ever since. On days off when he wasn't playing snooker and I wasn't playing football, we would jump in a car and travel round the country to different horse race meetings. Sometimes we'd have a big win, sometimes not, but we'd always have a laugh together. John's good company and was my best man when I married Jacqueline.

With John's wife being the sister of Duncan Ferguson's wife, there were obviously times when we would all be in each other's company. Duncan has been back on Merseyside for a bit now after living in Spain for a few years, and has been at Finch Farm working with the kids while trying to get his UEFA badges. From what I hear he has been doing very well. I wouldn't have necessarily thought of him as someone who would go into coaching, but, as he says himself, you can only lie on a beach for so long before you get bored.

He will be good at it because he is enthusiastic and he still has an aura about him. The kids will recognise that and look up to him because of it. If Duncan Ferguson tells you to work harder, or try doing something this way or that way, the youngsters will do it because they'll want to please him. That sort of relationship is important when you are a coach. It's all about respect.

Duncan has been to visit and has borrowed a couple of the training programmes I implemented during my time at Liverpool. He has taken them away to study, which shows he's eager to take on new ideas. But, having seen him close-up recently, I tell you he looks like he could still play. When he came to The Christie to visit, there was not an ounce of fat on him. He was in great shape.

So I have a network of wonderful friends who have helped me so much. Far more than they probably realise. But, even so, there is one person more than anyone else who has been my rock. It is difficult to put into words how much Jacqueline has done for me since I fell ill. Everything has been geared towards me since then and her life has been put on hold.

That is the thing about cancer. It does not just affect the sufferer, but so many other people as well. I don't know if I will make it through this illness and, consequently, her life is in limbo as well. I appreciate everything she's done for me so much. I hope she knows that.

There have been times that, as well as everything else, Jacqueline must have felt like she was my PA, organising my diary so that if people want to come and visit they can. It's nice that people consider me worthy enough to come and see because it's not as if I'm 10 minutes down the road. I suppose it shows I've left a positive mark on their lives, too.

I can take the kids to see Kenny or Moysey as a little treat, but it is important that Jacqueline has a break as well and finds the time to enjoy herself. She is always positive, looking forward to the future, keeping my spirits up, holding the family together, so it was brilliant to be able to go away to St Andrews in Scotland last October. Just the two of us. The League Managers' Association had set everything up for me. They had a deal with the old course hotel and paid for everything. We had a wonderful break. It was the first time we had been away since I was diagnosed, and it was the first occasion that alcohol had passed my lips as well.

I had actually vowed never to drink again when I became ill. It was not because I was told it would be harmful to my recovery. On the contrary, if I was staying in The Christie overnight then Samar, my consultant, would say it was alright for me to have a drink on the unit if I wanted one. That went for all the patients. I suppose it's a way of helping people to relax: lying on your hospital bed, can of lager in hand, watching whatever was on the television. Yet, the thought of drinking just never appealed to me. If friends came round they'd have a beer or a glass of wine, but I'd just have a cup of tea. I didn't feel like alcohol.

But up at St Andrews the food was fantastic, Jacqueline had a couple of cocktails and I had a couple of small glasses of red wine with my meal – and plenty of water. I suppose the trip was a reward for Jacqueline, not that she would feel like she needs 'rewarding', and not that two nights away in a posh hotel could ever repay what she has done for me. She is beautiful, caring, thoughtful, a wonderful mother and a brilliant wife. And I love her.

I must do because, one of the days we were up in Scotland, I joined her for a spa treatment and had something done to try and soothe my feet, which have swollen up really badly due to the steroids I am taking. We both came walking through in our fluffy robes ready for the treatment. If anyone had seen me, they would have thought: 'Look at that beaut there.' Spa treatments aren't normally 'me', so to speak...

It was just great to get away and we spent a few hours watching Liverpool draw with Manchester United in a nearby pub. This time I was back on the soft drinks, so I sat there sipping my Irn Bru as David de Gea denied Kenny and the lads what would have been a deserved league victory.

Part of the reason for going away was also to break the monotony of sitting in the house all the time. As a family, we have hardly been away together. You have to wait 12 months until after the transplant to travel long distances, but it would be a dream to take everyone away to Orlando or somewhere like that. The cost of the insurance for me would almost be as much as the holiday, of course – that's because I'm classed as 'high risk' these days – but sod that. Just to be away with everyone would be such a thrill. I'd maybe be able to lower the sun cream I'd have to wear, dropping down from factor 50 to something daring like 45.

I couldn't actually sit in the sun when I first came out of The Christie because I was susceptible to skin cancer, so I would sit with my sunglasses on, covered in the highest sun cream factor we could find. It becomes second nature after a while, but there was no chance of me picking up a tan.

So far the only time we have been away as a family was for a night at Carden Park in Cheshire, which was again fixed up for me by Sue and Emma from the League Managers' Association.

I was a bit embarrassed because we had not long come back from

St Andrews but, even though it was only for one night, just having everyone together meant it was a moment I treasured. I watched City stuff United 6-1 at Old Trafford with the boys before they went onto the driving range, and Jacqueline and Scarlet went for a spa.

Good times. Happy times.

Hopefully, there are more of those to come.

18

Fear And Hope

It was the middle of the night. I woke up with a fright, moved onto the edge of the bed and burst into tears. I was bawling. Sobbing uncontrollably. Everything that had happened to me, the fears that come hand in hand with living with cancer, came flooding out as I sat in the darkness worrying about the future.

Will I be around to see the kids growing up? What if I'm not around to walk Scarlet down the aisle when she gets married? What if this is the end? I was terrified, distraught and utterly beside myself. I cried that much that I woke Jacqueline up next to me and, as she attempted to comfort me, I confided in her what had exploded inside me: all of my fears, my concerns, my anxieties.

It wasn't that I was worrying about what was happening to me, but more about what might happen to my family if the worst came to the worst and I lost my battle with this terrible disease. How would they cope? How would they pay for things, even? My life has been in football, a game that everyone considers to be flushed with money these days, but I am not rich. What happens to the kids, to my wife, if I'm not around? How do they go on? The anxiety was choking me, closing around me. I couldn't see a way out. In an instant, I felt completely devoid of hope and gripped by this terrifying fear of what happens to those I would leave behind.

Jacqueline listened, took it all in, tried to soothe me and then did what she does best. She shrugged me out of myself. A few words knocked sense into me again. "Don't be so bloody stupid," she said. "Of course you will be here to do all that. And you'll do a lot more besides." She has that wonderful ability to fill me with optimism and confidence again, like she has throughout every day of the journey I have been on over the last 16 months. There have been so many times, not least on that occasion when I awoke in such blind panic, when I have realised I am so lucky to have her as my wife.

That night was the one real wobble I have had since I was diagnosed with cancer. I have certainly cried a lot more than once, when I've been sitting on my own maybe in the conservatory at home. There will be times when I sit there and think about what has happened and it'll bring a tear to my eye, but nothing like it did that night. But I think one episode like that in all the time that I have been ill, and with all the setbacks I have endured, isn't bad at all. In fact, it is good.

There are times when having cancer leaves you low and saps your spirit. Jacqueline will also tell you that there have been times when I have been an absolute bastard in terms of how I speak to her and how short my temper is with her and the kids. But I think the family has come to accept that it is not really me speaking. That it is to do with the medication that I am on and how tired I feel at times. I hope they realise that, anyway. And, for all those moments, there have been many more funny ones: times when, if you walked into a room, you'd find me laughing and joking like the next man.

There is no set way in which you should handle having cancer. There is no manual you collect from the consultant when you are diagnosed, saying: 'On Monday, laugh at 3pm. It'll make you feel better.' I have just tried to be as positive as I can throughout everything that has happened. I have tried to look forward, not backwards, and concentrate on what I can do as a patient.

Instead of that moment where I wonder if I will see the kids growing up, I'll look forward to taking the family to Orlando in Florida for a holiday. Things like that. Little goals and aims.

Even so, at times, it is still difficult. The easy part is telling yourself to be positive. The hard part is carrying it through. At times, the thoughts you have when you are first diagnosed come back into your head: 'Why me? Why?' But, with me, they don't linger nearly as long now as they once did.

It might seem strange, almost out of character perhaps, that I can be positive through this whole experience when my Liverpool career was so wracked with self-doubt. How can I front up to cancer when, at times, I shied away from wanting the ball at the club for whom I had always dreamed about playing?

But I think there always has to be an element of fear in whatever you do in order for you to perform to the maximum. If you asked the majority of top sportsmen or sportswomen, whether they be footballers or whatever, I think there is that small element of doubt, or fear, until you get out on the pitch and get your first touch or hit your first ball. Initially, for me, the fear extended to sitting in that changing room and doubting myself. Doubting whether I was good enough to do it. As I grew up, that balanced itself out. At Everton, there was the excitement of being in the dressing room and having the opportunity to go out and do what I'd always wanted to do.

Maybe I am able to be positive because I am older. Or maybe you have no choice but to be positive because, otherwise, it would get to you too much and overcome you. Certainly, they don't allow it to get you down in the hospital. I have two consultants, one who is completely straight laced – Adrian – and the other, Samar, who doesn't cover over anything but then quickly moves the conversation on to Liverpool Football Club. He's a massive fan and he always wants to know the ins and outs. If I'm honest, that helps. You take the bad news in, but you're not then sitting there dwelling on what you have just been told. You can't change it. It is what it is. You can't sugar coat it. It is just about getting on with it. I have to get on with it. Whether I have six months, or six years, or however long it is left, I just have to make the most of it.

* * * * * * * * * * * * * * * * *

I knew what was coming and I knew where I would find it. It would be right there for me on my pillow when I woke up, clumps of black hair serving as an early-morning reminder of the disease that I had. As if I needed one.

The first time I noticed my hair falling out as a side-effect of the chemotherapy was when I was staying at Milsoms in Ipswich, before my appointments at Addenbrooke's. And, despite being fully aware that this would more than likely happen, it was still difficult to get my mind around it. In fact, it was a complete shock.

One moment in particular sticks in my memory. I was back at home and, one morning, Hughie McAuley and his wife, Maria, were due to pop round for a cup of tea and a chat. I jumped into the shower, rubbed all my head wet and, as I took my hand away, clumps of hair came with it. It was literally coming out in chunks. I stared in the mirror, saw the bald patches appearing and panicked. I had worked with Hughie at Liverpool and Stockport and he had helped me out enormously as a coach. Over the years we've shared the same hopes, suffered the same disappointments and got to know each other inside out. I don't think there is anything I couldn't tell him.

But, despite all that, I didn't want him to see me like this. Normally, I would never wear a baseball hat, but I was desperate to preserve as much of my dignity as I could. I rummaged around the bedroom and found one, put it on and came down the stairs. I just sat there, not speaking. Hughie and Maria could tell something wasn't right because I couldn't bring myself to talk, but they didn't know what was on my mind. They probably just thought I was tired from all the treatment. But I knew what was happening under the cap and I was distant and monosyllabic as a result.

Looking back now, I think I wasted more energy on worrying about losing my hair than was really necessary. I understand why. Cancer had taken its toll on my body in so many ways that seeing my hair come out felt like one blow too many. It was a horribly visible confirmation that I was ill and I was suffering.

But, over time, I have had to learn to absorb the punches this disease has aimed at me and move on. So what if I was losing my hair? There are plenty of men my age who don't have my excuse. Theirs just falls out naturally. It actually became something we laughed about as a family. It was the only real way to deal with it, but that is an example of what I mean when I say about trying to be positive about things.

Jacqueline got in touch with her brother, who has his hair really short, and asked him to send the clippers up to the house. Well, the kids were soon demanding 'go faster' stripes down the side as I sat with a towel around my shoulders, waiting for Jacqueline to get to work. Thankfully, she didn't listen to them – no matter how much she might have wanted to play along with them at my expense – and just shaved it all really short. She made the point that I should regard losing my hair as a sign that I was getting better rather than getting worse. It was falling out because the treatment was working, and that is how I have tried to look at things ever since.

I have learned. During 2011, my hair started to fall out again because of the medication that I was on at the time. This time it didn't bother me. Why worry? I know it is going to grow back again eventually. I have never gone completely bald but, even if I did, I don't think it would affect me too much anymore. Not the same way as it would have in the past, anyway. The days when I would fret about what people would say are long gone. The people who know me, those who are my friends, aren't embarrassed when I am with them. They accept me for who I am, and what I'm going through. That means a lot to me.

Cancer has changed me, not just mentally but physically. When I look in the mirror, I still don't see myself. I don't recognise the man staring back. My face was always gaunt and pinched when I was a player, but it has been puffed up due to the steroids that I am on.

That's now. When I was first diagnosed, I weighed 96kgs. The lowest weight I have fallen to in the months since is 69kgs. I took a photograph of myself and, believe me, it doesn't look like someone who played at the top of the game for a decade. I am no longer the handsome athlete who won most of the medals that English football puts up for grabs!

But I have learnt to accept that. It is just part and parcel of what you go through with the treatment, and the people who matter to me have adopted that outlook as well. If that means I have no hair and my face is puffed up, if that means I can't walk too well and my co-ordination is all over the place because my feet are swollen, then it doesn't matter to them. That is what good friends do, and I have come to realise in recent months that I am fortunate in that respect. I have a lot of good friends, people I can rely on.

After leaving Addenbrooke's, I spent three weeks at The Christie in Withington, Manchester, and I have been back there every week since for treatment. I have had chemotherapy, a bone marrow transplant, about 40 lumbar punctures and, at one stage, I spent 12 days in there after developing Diabetes last September. The day I am told that I won't have to go back cannot come soon enough for me. I won't miss the waiting for treatment one bit. But the people who work there, on the other hand, have become such a big part of my life that not seeing them will be strange. They have been unbelievable: lifting my spirits, keeping me smiling, giving me the best care possible.

When I walk onto the ward, there is invariably a chant of "City, City, City" to greet me. Denise, Oonagh, Tracey, Dani and Adrian are the nurses who have helped to look after me, and they are all massive Manchester City fans. As I say to them: "Never mind, we can't all be perfect." But, increasingly these days with the way Roberto Mancini's side is playing, they have the final word. Imagine what it was like in there the week after City had beaten United 6-1 at Old Trafford in the 2011/12 season. Whatever you're thinking, multiply that by 100.

They had newspaper cuttings with the scoreline plastered over the walls in their little office and, if they could have put them on the ward, they would have. I walk in for my appointment and the first thing I hear is a lady called Denise singing: "We love you City, we do..." Fair play to them. They deserve to enjoy what's happening after so many years of being the butt of the jokes.

When Jacqueline and I drive over to The Christie there is inevitably that feeling of 'here we go again'. Then as soon as we get there, because they know us so well, there's a kiss and a hug. They're not like nurses anymore, more like friends. They'll complement Jacqueline on how she's looking, asking where she picked up those boots or that jacket. And they'll turn to me and say: "In your trackie, again Gary? You scruff." They like the banter, and I have to say it's good fun. I have to keep my wits about me if I'm to have the last word.

More seriously, though, if it wasn't for the patience and support that they have always shown me, I think my illness would have been far more difficult to cope with. That goes not just for me, but all the patients on the ward. I am sure the staff have their own stresses and worries in their own private lives. I am also sure that whatever they are paid, it does not come close to remunerating them for what a brilliant job they do. Some footballers will earn five, six, seven times more in a week than many of the nurses take home in a year. I suppose that is a symptom of the modern world we live in, but it can't be right, can it?

****

When I first went to The Christie I was having my blood checked every couple of hours, my blood pressure taken, my pulse read, my heart rate checked. The chemo is ordered from another site, as are the platelets and blood if you need them, and that is why the treatment can take time because you have to wait for the drugs to come to the ward. Rather than the chemotherapy being administered through a catheter through a vein in my arm all the time, a Hickman line was put into my chest and then to the top of the heart to ensure it goes directly there, rather than having to work its way around my body first.

Because my recovery was not progressing as well as the consultants had hoped, it wasn't long before it was mentioned that I might possibly need a bone marrow transplant. By November 2010, we were seriously discussing this option and, in the new year, I had my transplant.

I have taken on board so much medical terminology in the last year or so, that there becomes a point where your brain feels saturated. You have to push yourself to take everything in that the consultants are telling you like you did in the first place. That is partly because you implicitly trust the person who is telling you that a transplant is necessary, to the extent that you don't then need all the in-depth details. For that reason, I couldn't write a thesis on a bone marrow transplant – the procedure, the implications, the relevance even – but, basically, as I understood it, the bad cells in my bones had eaten away at the good ones and my body was failing. Or, it was in the process of failing.

Any disruption to the production of blood cells is serious because it affects your immune system. You can bleed out or bruise more easily, and you can also become starved of oxygen, which impacts on your organs. So I knew this was a significant step for me as I fought to regain my health, and pick up the pieces of my life again.

But, before the transplant itself could take place, I had to undergo total body radiation to eradicate all the existing bone marrow from my body. The sessions were time-tabled: half-an-hour in the morning, half-an-hour at night, over a period of four days and my body was wiped clean. The procedure isn't painful, just something else I knew I had to go through.

When the consultants explain that, with that amount of radiation involved, you are at a higher risk of getting tumours – more cancers, effectively – in years to come, you do think: 'Fucking hell.' But then you sign the piece of paper giving them the okay to plough ahead. Your faith in them cannot waver. They have to be right.

There was a lot of talk about where the bone marrow donor would come from. Germany was mentioned, the United States, too. But eventually they found a lady from Ireland who was a perfect match. You are not allowed to find out until a year after your transplant who your donor is, and only then if it has worked. I think that procedure is to protect the donor more than anything because if it hasn't worked, and something was to happen to whoever received it, it would make them feel terrible.

They had tested my brother Jeff, but there was only a one in four chance that he was going to be perfect match, or a 10-10 as they call it. The donors from the US and Germany were the same, so it was left to the lady from Ireland to come to my rescue. When we found the match, Jacqueline went out and bought some Irish balloons and she looked for a green wig. The only thing we were missing was the Guinness! That was all. Maybe that's why I get on so well with Roy Keane now, come to think of it!

But it is stupid things like that that keep you going. I'm going through this huge thing, fighting an illness that could claim my life but, for Jacqueline, going out and blowing up a load of green balloons helped keep her sane as well. Things like that take the edge off it all. You cling to anything you can in this situation, to be honest. Anything that will make you smile. Anything that allows you to appreciate humour. Anything that makes you feel properly alive.

I was due to have my transplant in January 2011 and, the night before, my consultant Samar came to see me. I didn't know this at the time but, when you have a bone marrow transplant, your DNA changes. Your fingerprints stay the same, but not your DNA. "Is there anyone you don't like," asked Samar, as we went through what would happen the next day.

"What do you mean?" I asked.

"Well, if you want to murder someone, do it now before your transplant because tomorrow you'll have a new DNA and no one will know it was you." I burst out laughing. Brilliant. Again, it was moment that lifted my spirits and eased the tension.

People like Samar, Adrian and professor Tim Illidge, who helped me out so much at the onset of the illness, are wonderful, wonderful people. Of course, you never want to have to meet them in such grave circumstances but, on the other hand, they are amazing.

Like Samar, Tim's life is football. One minute he'll be saving someone's life and the next he'll be telling you his perfect night out would be sitting on Graeme Sharp's table at Everton's end-of-season awards dinner. He knows the referee Mark Halsey, another cancer sufferer, and he'll show me photographs of himself with Sir Alex Ferguson, Moyesy and Sam Allardyce. I think he has enjoyed treating me in a way, a chance to spend some time with a former footballer.

There are two misconceptions about bone marrow transplants. The first is that it is an operation. It isn't, and I think it is actually more painful for the people who are donating the marrow than it is for the people who are receiving it. For me, it was like having a blood transfusion. I had two, 20-minute transfusions of stem cells which then work their way around the body, into the bones and then take affect by replenishing the bone marrow. The stem cells then take over the production of the blood cells.

The second misconception about bone marrow transplants is that once you have it, that's it. You're home and dry. Unfortunately, there is still a long way to go and, for me, the road has continued to contain many pitfalls. For starters, you have to think about getting immunised all over again. My thyroid was initially over-active after the transplant, which brought with it a whole host of side-affects. I became tired quickly, but then I didn't sleep well. I became irritable, too. I lost my appetite and I lost weight.

There was also a complication with graft-versus-host disease, in which the newly transplanted material attacked my body. My skin became dry – some sufferers can look like they are badly sunburnt – but, for me, the positive way to look at it was that it again showed that the new marrow was fighting and working. But those things, in all truthfulness, were minor.

It was in the August of 2011 when I suffered a far more significant setback.

19

The 'Big C'

I had instantly had a bad feeling about things when, as I went to see my other consultant, Adrian, I found his assistant, Ruth, in the room with him. 'She's not usually here', I thought to myself as I closed the door behind me. My mind drifted back to the meeting I'd had with Dr Fellows back when all this had started, when the lymphoma nurse was with him and he had said the cancer had spread to my spinal fluid.

There is no way you can dress up bad news and so Adrian just came out and said it. "The tests we have been doing show that there is evidence of some bad cancerous cells in the spinal fluid again," he said. There. Plain and simple. I was in serious trouble again.

My first reaction was to think: 'Shit.' For a few seconds I felt numb. This wasn't good. This wasn't what was supposed to happen. Then you naturally think, and start wondering if this is it. 'I am going to die.' Cue the tears.

Maybe because I had been through this before, when the bad cells were first detected, but after the initial shock I got my head around things. I won't pretend it was easy, but that's life for me now. Knock me down and I'll do my best to get back up again.

The spinal fluid leads up to the brain and so the treatment had to change. It had to become a lot more aggressive in trying to fight off the bad cells, but even then it is not as straightforward as that. Adrian explained that there is only so much of the treatment they could give me because of the toxicity of the drugs involved. I was warned that it could get to a stage where I couldn't have any more treatment. And, if I can't have any more treatment, then who knows what will happen? That is where I am today.

Travelling home in the car with Jacqueline that night my head was spinning but, once the situation had been explained to us, we both felt we had to be as honest as we could with the kids. Sitting Scarlet, Riley and Reece down on the sofa at home and explaining to them what the consultant had said was one of the hardest things I have ever had to do. There was no easy way to relay what the consultant had said. But there was no point trying to tell half-truths either. They deserved to know what the situation was.

I just said that if the treatment didn't work, I didn't know where I would stand. That if they couldn't give me any more treatment, then the truth is I had been told I might not be here in six months. I was crying, Jacqueline was crying. Seeing the kids dissolve into tears in front of me was heartbreaking.

Scarlet and Riley had a good cry, but Reece tried to tough it out. He wanted to be strong for his dad, but you could see his eyes were red raw. There isn't anything more you can say in that situation really. And then, amid the tears, another shaft of normality comes from nowhere. Jacqueline asked Riley what he was thinking about.

"About food," he said.

"Right, come on, let's go and get a Chinese then," we decided.

And that was it. We moved on. If they needed to ask anything or wanted to know anything, we told them to let us know. And, "Oh, do you want egg fried rice with your meal?"

The kids haven't particularly enjoyed coming to the hospitals. Addenbrooke's was different. It was so big, it had a Burger King in it and so it wasn't like a hospital in some respects. But The Christie has been largely off the map for them. I understand that. I don't think it is right to put them through that because you are never quite sure what you are going to see.

They tend not to ask that many questions, particularly when it comes to what is going to happen in the future. When I come back from the hospital each week, they always ask how it went and if I am okay. They just help out. You ask them to do anything and they'll help me. They do anything for me. We don't get into the nitty gritty of it, but they have grown up an awful lot while I've been ill. They have had to.

I love my kids and I'll continue to do anything for them, just as I will carry on battling every day for them. Spending time with them and Jacqueline is what drives me on and makes me determined to be strong again, to recover and keep going. But, to their enormous credit, they get on with their lives. Scarlet is turning into a young woman. She's at college studying fashion and is like her mum's clone. She loves to shop.

Reece is getting to an age where he is going to Liverpool games with Jacqueline's brother, Tony, and he'll go out after the match with him, too. I'm determined to take him myself soon. Father and son together at Anfield, just like it was when my dad first took me all those years ago. He is captain of his school team, and he plays on a Sunday for Tarleton Corinthians. He's 6ft and has turned into a good centre-half. Again, I'd like to think, a bit like his father.

It's funny because while he has gone towards Liverpool, Riley, as I say, is definitely more into Everton. He loves his trips to Finch Farm to watch the players train.

Riley plays football too and is the vice-captain of his age group with Tarleton Corinthians. Unfortunately, I don't get to see him and Reece playing as much any more. I used to go and watch every Sunday without fail, but I find it difficult walking to the pitches, which are on the far side of the park and, in autumn and winter especially, I also have to make sure that I don't leave myself open to infection. Catching colds or flu these days could have huge implications because my immune system is still quite low.

I had stopped having to have the lumbar punctures, but the re-emergence of the bad cells meant I went back on to that course of treatment. At least I knew what was coming my way. At least the fella who does it, Kaz, is top class.

Basically, a needle goes into my back and they withdraw a 20ml sample, before another needle goes in and the chemo is then administered. It goes straight into the spinal column and that then transports it up to, into and around the brain, and tries to kill off any of the bad cells that are there.

That sounds terrifying – the reality is merely unpleasant.

I used to Tweet when I came out of hospital because I found it was the best way of letting everyone know how my treatment was going. I would never really pass comment on football. It was more just: "Been to the hospital, everything okay today." Stuff like that. Little updates. However, I closed down my account not long after I had been told the bad cells had come back because someone Tweeted a rumour that they had heard I was terminally ill, and had only had six months to live.

It wasn't true, but people don't realise just what effect that has on the people close to me. As soon as someone sends that sort of message, they will invariably forget about it. They move on, getting on with their lives. It isn't like that for us. I understand that they are not being malicious, but so many people are on Twitter these days that everything becomes fact straight away.

Jacqueline and I had to sit the kids down when they came home from school once again and tell them not to believe it. Moments like that really test you. They test your patience because you immediately become angry, but as long as the people I love know the truth, that is the most important thing. The bad cells coming back is just another hurdle that has been placed in front of me. And I'll do everything to make sure I clear it.

* * * * * * * * * * * * * * * * *

It has taken time for me to get my head around things, but to me the 'Big C' is no longer simply about cancer. It is about choice. And it is about making decisions that will positively affect my life and the lives of those around me whom I love.

This is a message I want to get across to other people in all walks of life, not just in sport. And, even, not just those who find themselves in a similar position where they have been struck down by this illness.

Because I have not worked for the past year and a half, I have to think about ways of bringing in money, supporting my family and paying the mortgage just like everyone else. So I initially came up with the idea of going into various football clubs and making a presentation to the youngsters there about how the choices they make in their careers today will affect the rest of their lives.

Hopefully, clubs would look to get their first team involved further down the line but, at first, I planned to speak to scholars, the Under-18s and reserve squads. I am wary of taking it any lower than the Under-16s because I think what we talk about could be upsetting for that age group. Over the course of a couple of days, I could give the presentation maybe four times to the various different groups.

Of course, it would be up to each individual person sitting in the classroom whether they wanted to listen to me or not. Whether they wanted to take in what a footballer, whom I accept many of them will never have seen play, is going on about.

Maybe the presentation would be delivered after the players have had their lunch. They've trained all morning, they're tired and they know they could be resting and relaxing in the changing room instead of being sat in front of me. So, for the next hour, do they listen? Or do they treat me as background noise and simply doze off? Do they take on board what I am saying, from the minute they walk out of the door and set foot back on the training pitch, to try and put a few things into practice, or not? It's their choice.

I would hope people would listen to what I have to say and be keen to interact with me. How do you cope with not playing on a Saturday? How do you cope with rejection from your club? I can offer insight into matters like that. What type of people do you surround yourself with? I would touch on all that and bring my own experiences into it.

You can't make great decisions all the time. It is impossible. And you may make decisions that you think are great at the time, but when you look back on them you're not so sure. Obviously, some decisions are sometimes made for you in life as well.

I did a course a couple of years ago with Mark Proctor, the former Middlesbrough midfielder, and he told me that he knew for a fact that they had bid £2.5m for me when I was at Liverpool.

That was the first I had ever heard of that, and it's only years later that you wonder about how your career could have been different. Presumably, it wasn't enough money, which is flattering in many respects, and given Graeme's attitude towards me presumably the bid came in when Kenny was in charge.

But it was strange to learn, years later and second hand, that another club had tried to sign me. My career could have gone a completely different way.

There is nothing major in my career I wish I had done differently.

Joining Everton was a controversial decision at the time and the stick I took was horrendous, but it paid off for me. It's written down in the history books as having done so anyway. Gary Ablett: the only player to claim FA Cup winner's medals with both Liverpool and Everton.

I suppose there will be people who say my decision to stand up for myself at Liverpool when I was a coach under Rafa was a poor choice. It cost me my job, after all. It cost me a lot of money, and the chance to work at a fantastic club.

But I have my principles and I chose to stand by them. I chose to speak my mind. That's who I am. And I don't regret anything. Again, these are things I can talk about, and maybe what I've learned will stand others in good stead.

Basically, the presentation is ready to go when I am ready to do it. It is about feeling well enough and having the energy to go through with it. When I was first ill, I would be waking up some mornings at 5am. I couldn't sleep, I couldn't get comfortable. So I would tip-toe downstairs and sit in the front room with a stopwatch and time myself giving my presentation. The first time I did it, it lasted 25 minutes. 'Oh my God,' I thought. 'This isn't going to work.'

But the more confident I became, the more I remembered about my career and my life. The more I practised, the longer it ran for. I stretched it out to 55 minutes and that is without any interaction or feedback from the audience. That works.

I am looking forward to delivering it, to be honest. It would begin with some clips of me scoring and playing for Everton, and then would head straight into the illness. The idea is to shock people. I go from being this strong, athletic footballer to basically being transformed into a bag of bones at one point, and then I come out the other side. Someone who is facing up to the reality of living with cancer and trying to be positive about it.

I am comfortable now getting up in front of people because I have done that for the last seven or eight years. When you first stand up in front of a dressing room of 20 players, it can be nerve-wracking. You want to be liked, but you don't want to be seen as a soft touch. You want to be interesting without being over the top.

So walking into a room full of strangers won't bother me and, if there are more than 20 people at each presentation, then so much the better. That would mean I am reaching out to more people and discussing the choices we all make.

The feedback I have had on the idea has been positive. I want to reach out to the Football Association and the Professional Footballers' Association, while the Premier League has said it will help me with contacting clubs.

I have been in to see Frank McParland at Liverpool and he has been supportive. Everton always back me to the hilt. The League Managers' Association, who have been brilliant with me also, put me in touch with Jeremy Snape, the former England and Leicestershire cricketer who has also been a member of the South Africa cricket team's backroom set-up.

He has his own company, Sporting Edge, which does a lot of motivational and team-bonding courses at a corporate level, and he thinks my story has a really powerful message to send to people.

With Jeremy's help, there has been interest from a hockey club in the south of England and that has given me the confidence that there is an appeal beyond football's boundaries.

Remember, 2012 is going to be a huge year for athletes with the Olympics coming to London and I genuinely feel that I could get across a positive message to competitors in this country, that this is their chance of a lifetime.

Schools could get involved, community colleges, rugby clubs, everyone.

So it is really down to me now.

It is down to me to regain my health, regain my energy and go out and about and tell people my story.

That is the choice I have made and, every day, when I wake up, that aim is at the forefront of my mind.

My life has changed since I contracted the 'Big C,' but my choice is that I won't let it beat me.

Gary Ablett, December 6, 2011

Epilogue

A Light Shines On

My husband, Gary, passed away in the early hours of January 2, 2012.

The day of his funeral in the Anglican Cathedral in Liverpool, it was cold and miserable. I remember thinking as we drove in, 'I just hope it doesn't rain.'

As we got onto the Dock Road leading to the city centre, it started looking brighter but by the time we got to cathedral and went in for the service, it was overcast once again.

"I hope the sun comes out," I said.

"Then I know Gary will be okay and happy."

The turnout for Gary was overwhelming.

So many people attended, for which I am truly thankful, although I don't think I took everything in.

I remember recognising Reece's schoolteacher among the congregation, but for much of the time I was just thinking of Gary and not even looking up because I knew I would get even more upset.

Then, one moment in particular will stay with me forever.

The cathedral is such a beautiful building and I remember looking towards Reverend Canon Henry Corbett when he was speaking. It was then that, from nowhere, the sun starting shining through the huge stained glass window and lighting up all the colours.

It got brighter and brighter, illuminating the service, and then faded again. It was amazing and that was enough.

I know that ray of sunshine was Gary. He was saying, 'I'm here. Love you, love the kids.'

Since the service, so many people have mentioned that to me. I got a text from Brendan Rodgers, the Swansea manager who was reserve-team coach at Chelsea when Gary was in charge of Liverpool reserves, saying how fitting it was. That Gary brightened up people's lives.

This will sound bizarre to some people but when Gary was in hospital, I would come home and the house would feel empty. Since he has passed away, I don't get that eerie feeling any more. I feel him around me.

That first night, my mum, me and the kids were sat together, just talking and I was saying: 'I hope he lets me know he is okay'.

On the conservatory door, I had a wreath that had been hanging there from before Christmas.

As we spoke, the wreath just dropped to the floor. We looked at each other and even the kids said, "Oh my God, that's dad."

The hook was still in the door.

Several weeks on, it is remembering moments like this that help myself and the kids to keep going.

And, of course, Bella the bulldog.

Back in August 2011, when Gary was told the cancerous bad cells had come back again, he had wanted to get a dog for the kids.

I'd talked him out of it at the time because there was so much going on that it didn't seem the right moment to start looking after a puppy.

We'd go on the internet, look at the different breeds and the idea was to get one the following summer when Gary was stronger again.

It was Christmas Eve when Bella came into our lives. I'd been toying with booking a holiday for everyone as Gary's Christmas present when one of the kids suggested getting a dog. The next thing Scarlet was on the iPad and had found two pups in Preston, which is just a few miles down the road from where we live.

It was always the intention just to go and have a look, but when you see this beautiful puppy staring back at you and your heart melts, it is hard to say 'no'.

They brought this little, seven-week old bulldog pup through and the kids and I were all like: "Oh my God." That was it. Decision made.

I went off to the bank to get the money and Scarlet went into Marks & Spencer to get a lovely, pink dog blanket.

I can't remember exactly where the name Bella came from. Someone just said it. But it fits perfectly. As soon as I put her on Gary's bed, there was a huge smile on his face.

I'm so glad we got Bella because there was definitely a bond between them. She would go in and see Gary and sit on the bed. I knew it made Gary happy.

Every now and again, Bella will go into the bedroom and have a little sniff around, expecting Gary still to be there.

****

We had always dealt positively with Gary's illness.

When he was first diagnosed, he had battled and fought and he did so well. Everything was really positive. We didn't let things affect us too much. We are a close family and we helped each other. We took things in, dealt with them in our own way and moved on.

Even when the bad cells came back, we said: "We'll cope."

I always remember the nurses at The Christie saying that at some point we would need help. You listen and take it in, but I never thought it would come to that.

It was a couple of weeks before Christmas that Gary was due to go in to hospital and have a lumbar puncture and his fortnightly review. He was taking water tablets at the time. He was also on steroids and his feet were swollen up as a result of the medication. He had difficulty walking.

"I don't want to go," he said. I rang The Christie and they said, "Fine. No problem. Come in tomorrow."

Gary didn't want to go in the next day. I put it down to the steroids because they had changed him. He wasn't himself. He was sleeping a lot and spent a lot of time in bed. Either myself, or one of the kids, would always be with him. There was always someone there to keep him company. When it came to Christmas, we brought him his dinner on a tray in the bedroom.

It was around that time that Gary's condition deteriorated.

I know 100 per cent that it wasn't because he didn't want to fight on. I know that. I saw every day how brave Gary was. How courageous he was. How unselfish he was. How positive he was in setting himself little goals like looking forward to a holiday or something like that.

The truth is that I just think he had reached the stage when he couldn't fight anymore. He didn't have the strength.

The nurses who came to see him said he seemed to be in a lot of pain. But one of the things about Gary throughout his entire battle for health was that he never, ever said he was in pain. He would just say, "I can't get comfortable."

That was it, and he would never take any painkillers.

Around this tume, one of the nurses asked: "On a level of 1-10, how bad is it, Gary?"

"Nine," he said.

That was just how Gary was. He would tell the nurses, but try and protect me by saying he was fine so that I wouldn't worry as much. Again, thinking of others instead of himself.

****

What really helped me on the day he passed away was seeing all the messages we received on Twitter. I was up until 2am the next morning reading them.

We all think our family and husbands are special, but the response has been amazing. It was overwhelming and a huge comfort for all of us. Everyone has lost someone they love at some point and a lot of people were saying they'd lost loved ones to cancer. I started responding to them and it really helped me.

In some senses, the support we have received has been difficult to get my head around.

The thing about Gary was that he would never really go into Liverpool city centre. He looked to keep a low profile, mainly because of the reaction he received when he moved from Liverpool to Everton. He never wanted to put the kids in a position whereby someone might say something.

So the out-pouring there has been since Gary died seems unreal. Where has it all come from?

We kept out of the way and then, for all this to happen... you do scratch your head.

I know it is sincere and I know that everyone means it. Maybe the truth is that it has taken something really sad to happen for people to realise how they felt about Gary all along.

****

People have said to me, "I don't know how you have coped." But a lot of the time I know it was because I had Gary. As long we had each other, then we would be alright.

For all the time Gary was ill, we both missed the life we had before when we took so much for granted I suppose.

You wonder how the kids are going to cope. They get upset at times. There are times we all get upset and you sit and think about the things you miss.

But we are a close family and I am proud of the way the kids have handled everything. They have had to grow up an awful lot over the course of the last 20 months.

When Gary was the manager at Stockport, someone once said they'd seen me walk past a room and when I disappeared out of sight, Scarlet appeared before walking past. Then Reece. Then Riley. I was like the mother hen with my three little chicks in line behind me.

That hasn't changed. They are doing alright.

Reece is the comedian and he keeps us all laughing. But I read little Tweets from him and I know how strong and how brave he is being as well.

Riley, too. He is my little comforter. The one I get my cuddles off. He couldn't wait to score his first goal for Tarleton Corinthians after Gary passed away so that he could point up to the sky to his daddy.

Scarlet is fantastic. She watched all the tributes on Sky Sports when Gary died, and took it upon herself to text the likes of Alan Hansen, Jamie Carragher and Ian Rush just to say thanks for their support.

I didn't know she had done that, she did it off her own bat. She has been an absolute star.

Scarlet was a daddy's girl. She idolized him, and she is now on a mission. Gary always had an idea to open a clothes agency whereby footballers' wives would donate old clothes, be it a pair of shoes, a dress, a jumper or something like that, and some of the money would go to charity.

Scarlet is determined to get it up and running. We have spent weekends driving around Liverpool and Crosby looking for shops to rent, and she has really got the bit between her teeth. She wants to make a go of it and do it in her dad's name. If I know Scarlet, then no one will stop her. We have had a meeting about it with Sue McKellar from the League Managers' Association, who has continued to offer her support to the family.

Sue and LMA chief executive Richard Bevan are just some of the people I have to thank. It is difficult to know where to start, but I would like to pay tribute to The Christie Hospital and the staff on the HTU out-patients and those on the ward for their patience, understanding and selflessness.

To Ipswich Hospital and Addenbrooke's Hospital for the care they offered to Gary; to Tarleton District Nurses; to Ipswich Town Football Club, the players, staff and CEO Simon Clegg; to the staff at Everton FC, in particular Mike Dickinson, and Liverpool FC.

Thanks also to Roy Keane for his unbelievable support, friendship and kindness during Gary's illness and since. You have been amazing.

And to Ste and Janette Jones; Matt Jackson and his family; Vinny and Tracy Samways and family; Thomas Fairclough and Reverend Canon Henry Corbett for their support.

I would like to thank both mine and Gary's parents and both our families. Ann Ablett, my sister-in-law, for holding my hand and helping me through the funeral arrangements with Hardman's Funeral Directors and Liverpool Anglican Cathedral.

My three amazing nieces – Louise, Toni and Raychel Moore – and Paul Joyce for running the boys to watch Liverpool training and helping Gary write this book. I know that reminiscing about everything he crammed into his career during the writing of this book was both enjoyable for him and also therapeutic.

Also, thank you to the vets and nurses at Rufford Veterinary Group for looking after Bella so well.

To everyone who sent cards, letters, flowers, donations, tweets and texts: Thank you. To all our close friends who were always there for us, and to all the new friends I have made throughout such a difficult time, your support is greatly appreciated.

The children and I would just like to say from the bottom of our hearts: thank you for everything. Your kind words and amazing support has really helped us through a heartbreaking time.

****

A few weeks before he first fell ill, Gary mentioned that he wanted to do something to help others. He suggested that he would like to use his name and what he had achieved in football to set up a charity or a foundation.

This came totally out of the blue and at the time we didn't think too much about it. We were getting on with our lives as a family and we didn't take it any further. What happened next was that Gary received the shock news he was suffering from non-Hodgkin's lymphoma.

The idea was forgotten about while he battled the illness. It was never mentioned again because Gary was always positive and assumed that he would get better, and there would be time to look at things like this at some stage in the future.

It is only now that I look back after everything that happened and realise that Gary planted a seed of an idea, and that it is up to us to make sure that it becomes a reality.

We are so proud of what Gary achieved as a footballer and who he was as a person.

We are also so grateful for the support we have received, and see this as an opportunity to give something back and leave a lasting legacy in his name.

It is all at an early stage. We have made a few enquiries and had some help from various people who have had experience of setting something like this up.

We don't know yet exactly what form it will take, but we know that we are determined and want something positive to come out of what has happened.

We know that's what Gary would have wanted.

Jacqueline Ablett, March 2012

I

—

To Dad

The following passages were put together by Scarlet, Reece and Riley and read out at the service for Gary at the Anglican Cathedral...

Dad was one the nicest people in the world, he always put others before himself, especially us and our incredible mum. We are so proud of the amazing man he was and even more proud of how brave he was for the last 16 months.

Not once did we ever hear him ask why this was happening to him or moan about the situation he was in, because that's the type of person he always was, he picked himself up and carried on.

Two things we will remember from the past 16 months is he always kept that sense of humour throughout, it wasn't that long ago he was bouncing off the walls because of the steroids and shuffling round the living room to LMFAO and Chris Brown thinking he was dead cool!

And it also wasn't that long ago he was wanting to give those group of girls a piece of his mind for giving his princess grief.

Secondly, that massive gorgeous smile that stayed with you right up until your final days.

I could go on for years about how amazing he was but I won't, I'll just say – 'Dad, you were my best friend and I will never ever find anyone that will come close to being half the best friend you were to me. You were always there for me no matter what, whether it was problems with friends or when I was just feeling sick. I'm gutted you'll no longer be here to give me a cuddle or even to make fun of me'.

But now you're finally at peace and no more suffering, I know I'm going to spend the rest of my life hurting inside but I'm also going to spend the rest of my life loving you and remembering what a super dad, husband, friend and all-round person you were.

So, Dad, behave up there (I know you won't) and carry on looking after us because I know you're still here.

Anyway I'll see you later pal...

Love always, your little princess Scarly-Warly

Well, Dad, it only feels like yesterday that we were going to the Liverpool games every week and I was sitting there pulling faces to myself thinking no-one was watching me, and you were still going on about that moment two or three years after.

I remember mum used to take me to football every Saturday and I still hadn't scored a goal but the first game you took me to I managed to score a screamer. The Ablett magic must have rubbed off on me for that one game, I'm still trying to get that magic back.

One of the last things I'm going to remember is when we were sitting in your hospital room playing some puzzle game that Roy gave you and I couldn't complete one of them, not even the easiest one.

TO DAD

Then later that night I got a text off you saying 'puzzle 2 completed' and in about half an hour I had 15 texts off you saying you'd completed a new puzzle. Well Dad, or 'Big G' as I prefer, I'm already missing you a lot and I know I'm going to miss you a lot more but I'll never forget everything you've done for me and I promise I won't let anyone else forget you.

Love you 'Big G'.

II

—

Tributes

Just some of the many comments about Gary that appeared in the press and some that have been written for this book...

Big brother, I hope that I can find the words to pay you the tribute that you deserve. You are one of the few people I know who lived their dream. It wasn't handed to you on a plate, it was through hard work and dedication that you achieved that dream. Playing football was the only thing that you ever wanted to do from way back to our kickabouts in the back garden when we were kids.

You should be proud of your achievements as a professional footballer but, more importantly, as a man. To me your biggest achievement was as a loving husband to Jacqueline and father to five beautiful children, Scarlet, Reece, Riley, Joshua and Fraser, and you should be proud of them all. I know you will be watching over them somewhere.

You faced the biggest battle of your life over the last 18 months and showed great courage and bravery that made me prouder than I have ever been of you. I always thought that you would beat your illness because you were my big brother and you always won. Sadly this was the one battle you couldn't win, and now there is a big empty space in the lives of the people who loved you the most.

My biggest regret is that I was not more a part of your life, as I always thought that you would be there and there would always be tomorrow. Now that you are gone, those days will never come and all I am left with are my memories of you and the thoughts of never seeing that big smile again.

A friend gave me this verse after you passed. It sums up how I feel and how I hope everyone will remember you this way when they think of you:

You can shed tears that he has gone
or you can smile because he has lived.
You can close your eyes and pray that he'll come back
or you can open your eyes and see all he's left.
Your heart can be empty because you can't see him
or you can be full of the love you shared.
You can turn your back on tomorrow and live yesterday
or you can be happy for tomorrow because of yesterday.
You can remember him and only that he's gone
or you can cherish his memory and let it live on.
You can close your mind, be empty
or you can do as he'd want, smile and go on.

I'm so glad that I had the chance to tell you how proud I always was to have you as my brother and that you are, and always will be, my hero. But most of all, I'm glad I told you that I loved you.

God bless, until we meet again.

(Your loving brother Jeff)

Sam and I are so sorry for your loss; we both cherish the memories of our time spent with you and Gary. I have always believed in life that you are meant to meet certain people, if only briefly, who have come to teach you something important. Little did I know that when I first met Gary, he would teach me life's greatest lesson.

It was a lovely, sunny day sitting on Mitchell Field (New York) chewing the fat, at first about footy! But soon we discussed life. Gary said something that started a change in me. He told me that he had found the secret to happiness in life. For him it was family – and how right he was. Gary lit a spark that made me think about what I really wanted. Without meeting him, I truly believe I would not have found the happiness I have with my own family. For which I will be eternally grateful.

Friends have been asking me about Gary and I have told them that what they have read about the man I found to be true. Above all things that I admired about him, the things that shone through were his honesty and dignity. I was privileged to call him a friend.

And as hope fades into the world of night, through shadows falling out of sight and memory and time, don't say we have come to journey's end. As the pale moon rises across the sea, the ships have come to carry you home. And dawn will turn to silver clouds, a light on the water. White shores are calling you, but we will meet again.

Always in our prayers.

(Friends Markco, Sam and Yanni)

This is my third attempt at writing this tribute and despite wanting everything to be perfect, I keep making mistakes. I keep wondering what great things everyone is saying and how eloquently they will express Gary's character. So, I am going to say it as I first saw it. Gary was an ordinary man.

I never knew him during his playing career but got to know him during the 15 months before he died. He seemed so ordinary, he loved all sports and the first time I met him he showed a very normal male ability to flick between three different sports channels on TV at the same time. He asked if I could help him to develop some of his stories into a keynote speech for school, sport and corporate audiences. At first I was just happy to help and then as I listened more, the real themes began to emerge.

I was beginning to link stories of overcoming adversity and his courage to choose his own path. I heard of his dad's motorbike trips to matches and his headmaster's 'poor' advice to avoid football. I heard of a youngster rubbing shoulders with the Liverpool greats, and then choosing to swap that life for a blue shirt with the team up the road. I heard of a man whose dignity and integrity shouted louder than his words, a passion for helping others and a man whose family always came first. Each time I drove away from Gary's house, I had a deeper and more privileged insight into the way Gary's life had unfurled. But that was just the point: it hadn't unfurled, he had made a series of brave choices which had enriched his life. We called his presentation "The Big C" but it was not about cancer, it was about choice, and Gary demonstrated in high definition that whatever happens to us, our power lies in our choice of attitude.

This is when I realised my biggest mistake – Gary Ablett was anything but an ordinary man.

Although Gary never narrated his presentation in public, this book carries this most powerful of legacies. His courage to choose the right response in the toughest of life's challenges is a lesson which anyone who met Gary will never forget.

(Ex-England cricketer and Sporting Edge
founder Jeremy Snape)

First and foremost he was a really good guy, a terrific servant to the club as a player and as a coach and it's a really sad day for everyone at Liverpool, but the people who matter most in this situation are his family and our thoughts are with them.

I'm sure everyone at Everton speaks the same as everyone at Liverpool does and that speaks volumes for Gary, the respect he has at both places. He was a top guy and a top professional in the way he went about his work. He was enthusiastic and all the players who worked under him for the reserves and the first team learned a lot off him.

I only worked with Gary in certain sessions, but I could see that he was a very good coach. What I remember from Gary was how he conducted himself; he always had a smile on his face and was enthusiastic and that rubbed off on me personally and the rest of the players.

(Liverpool captain Steven Gerrard)

No sooner had I got into the team than I realised, 'hang on a minute, it's not going to be long before this guy is going to be breathing down my neck.'

That guy was Gary and I knew he was a threat to my dreams at Liverpool even if his versatility meant he could play in other positions, not just left-back.

We were rivals, but above that we were mates. And that counted for more. If we could help each other out we would. When I came over to Liverpool from Ireland, Gary was one of lads who was friendly towards me and his family were very good to me. That helped me enormously and I will never forget that.

I knew he was a good guy, one of the best, simply by how his family was. Liverpool was a harsh environment at that time. The club was setting the bar not just in England, but we knew if the European ban hadn't been in place we would have been the best in Europe too. Gary can be proud then of what he achieved in a Liverpool jersey because you had to be good enough to play alongside the stars and he was a good player with a great attitude.

Getting up to speak in the Anglican Cathedral at Gary's funeral is one of the hardest things I have had to do. I used the words "genuine" and "sincere" because Gary was, but he had so many other qualities too. Honest, humble, loyal. I'm still in shock now at his passing and can't believe he has gone.

(Liverpool team-mate Jim Beglin)

He was a lovely guy and he was quite unassuming – everyone loved him. It is such a shock, even though we knew he was ill. I texted him on December 7 to go and see him and have a cup of tea and he texted back to say he had a doctor's appointment but wished me a merry Christmas, and said he would see me in the new year.

Then we get the news this morning and we are absolutely stunned and cannot believe this has happened. Talking to two or three ex-Liverpool players we are all distraught because we all thought he was fine and recovering. (To die at) 46 years of age is absolutely tragic. Each and every one of us is stunned by the news.

He came into the dressing room when Liverpool had one of the great teams and he was right in there because he was a top-class player as well. If he had joined Liverpool in the late '70s or early '80s he would have been a permanent fixture.

He was a dedicated, consummate professional but he was right at the top of the tree. I had a couple of great centre-back partnerships at Liverpool and he was as good as anyone. I played with him when he was on the left-side of defence and he made it easy for me. As soon as he stepped into the Liverpool side I knew he was a top-class player."

(Liverpool legend and team-mate Alan Hansen)

We knew Gary had been ill for quite a while. I heard recently it was bad news and it would be a matter of time. He fought it for a long time. That is the type of person he was. He was a super fellow. It is a sad day and I am stunned. He was just 46.

He was a tremendous worker and a good defender. I took him to Sheffield United as well. He was a consistent player. He had a great career in football and made a big contribution to the game.

(Former Everton manager Howard Kendall)

Gary was a lovely, lovely guy who was liked by everyone. I don't think anyone will have a bad word to say about him.

He was a classy defender and had decent quality going forward as well and he was not dirty in any way. But because of his understated way he was maybe under-rated by many people. It says something that I enjoyed playing against him even in the Merseyside derby – which is one of the most stressful games in world football – because he was just such a nice guy. I'm shocked and saddened.

(Everton team-mate Pat Nevin)

He was a great person. I knew him when he was here as a coach and he did a fantastic job, winning the league in his second season. He had a great rapport with the lads, particularly the younger ones.

There are not many people who can cross the divide between Everton and Liverpool like he did, both as a player and coach; no one at either club has ever had a bad word to say about him and that's evidence of the high esteem he's held in.

You can see what a great coach he was from the response he got from the players and the job he did here; we took him from Everton so that says a lot about him and how good he was.

When you speak to the younger lads like Martin Kelly and Jay Spearing and see them in the first team now, you see the impact he's had on their careers and he should take a great deal of credit for their development, along with the staff in the academy.

He was a great player for Liverpool and for Everton; he won the FA Cup with both teams. That will probably never happen again and that's a great achievement. He played in a great Liverpool side with the likes of Barnes, Beardsley and Aldridge and to be involved in that was something special. When he went to Everton he was part of the great side they had there with Joe Royle and the 'dogs of war' team.

He was a great bloke and he always had a smile on his face; that's how I'll remember him, great to be around. Even when you'd see him after he had the illness, he still had that bubbliness about him, trying to keep spirits high. That's a great testimony to him as a person. He'll be sorely missed by everyone but most of all his family.

(Liverpool vice-captain Jamie Carragher)

He was my boot boy, around 1981, and my first memories of him are as a really nice lad, who was very polite and respectful of the senior pros. He was a tall, thin, gangly lad but he was a great runner. One of the lads nicknamed him Seb, after Sebastian Coe.

I think I had left when he broke into the first team, but it was obvious he was always going to get there. He knew he had to work hard to make it, and that is what he did. He had lots of pace to recover and he was very good on the ball. He was a good team-mate, you could never have enough Gary Abletts in your team. He was a real gentleman.

(Liverpool team-mate Mark Lawrenson)

Late, late on in the game [1995 FA Cup semi-final] he made an unbelievable run to set up one of the goals. The game was already won but he ran almost the length of the pitch when he didn't need to and that just about summed him up.

We had some good years playing at Everton together. He was so brave to make the move having been so successful at Liverpool. It can't have been easy to come to Everton but he was successful there as well.

I was surprised how good he was and I shouldn't have been. It's very often the case that with unsung heroes it's easy not to give them the credit they deserve, but I saw what a good player he was. He had a wonderful left foot, was fantastically cool and a natural athlete. He was versatile, could play anywhere on the left or at centre-half and never complained about where he was asked to play. He was a very under-stated person and such a genuine, generous man. He had a great sense of humour and was just very giving. It was a pleasure to play with him.

(Everton team-mate Barry Horne)

It is very sad news. I will remember Gary as a really good footballer. He was a very good reader of the game, a good passer and always used the ball well. He did everything to the best of his ability. He was very composed and had a sweet left foot.

Off the field he was a quiet guy, a family man. He loved the fact he had made it as a footballer – that was all he had ever wanted to do.

(Liverpool team-mate Jan Molby)

I enjoyed playing alongside Gary and I enjoyed his company. His great characteristic was how humble he was. He'd come from Liverpool and Everton and won trophies, but you'd never have known it.

He was a really nice bloke. When something like this happens to a person like Gary everything else in football pales into insignificance.

You hear nonsense about players now but Gary had seen it, done it and bought the T-shirt and remained down to earth, a normal lad. We were old stagers coming to the end of careers when we joined Birmingham but there was a pride about us, we wanted to do our best and achieve something with the club.

Gary was a steady-Eddie type but an excellent defender. He had a lot of quality and drew on all his experience and I think the Birmingham fans appreciated how good a player he was.

Gary had that dry sense of Scouse humour. But he was also tight. After a while he suggested we use my car to come down in all the time, but he'd drive. Basically it was a case of my car, my petrol, my money – he wanted to save himself a few bob! It's a sad loss and all our thoughts are with Gary's family.

(Birmingham City team-mate Steve Bruce)

It is a big shock. Obviously we know Gary was ill. It is a really sad day. He was good at everything he did as a player. He went into coaching, stamped his personality onto that and was doing a very good job.

(Former Liverpool manager Roy Evans)

Gary was a really versatile player, somebody who would play anywhere the manager asked him. The fact he played for both Liverpool and Everton says something about how good he was as a player.

He summed up what Liverpool people are all about. He gave 100 per cent to the team and my favourite memory of him was after the 1989 FA Cup final. He was so proud to win something for the team.

He was a very knowledgeable football man, too. He was not a shouter and a raver, he was more of a coach. He knew a lot about the game and he could see potential in young players – a skill in itself.

Off the pitch, he was the perfect gentleman. He had a lovely family, which he brought up really well, and he was such a respectable person. If he could help you with anything, he would.

(Liverpool team-mate Ian Rush)

Gary impressed me the first time I met him as a 14-year-old. He was a member of Liverpool Schools' Under-15 team and, although he was a year younger than the other members of the team, he had a really professional way about him. It was as if he was the senior member of the squad and he assumed the role of 'leader by example'.

As the years went on I continued to have contact with Gary through Merseyside Schools' football and as a young apprentice at Liverpool, where he played alongside a couple of other young hopefuls, Chris and Mark Seagraves, whom I had taught. He was the stand-out member of the reserve team and carried himself in a way that suggested he would go on to become a player of some note in the future – and so he did!

When he eventually went to play in America, after a very successful career here in England, we lost touch, but on his arrival back in England we met up at one of Everton's FA Youth Cup matches. He was the same modest and respectful young man that I knew but had not seen for some time. He now had his sights set firmly on coaching and was very quickly working his way through his awards.

During the time he worked with our young players at Everton he was the perfect role model and influenced them in ways that he didn't even realise. More recently as he was engaged in his battle with non-Hodgkin's lymphoma he was absolutely the same Gary Ablett that he had always been and, if anything, more humble than ever.

Gary had a profound effect on many people during his difficult times as well as his good times and he will continue to do so long after his passing. He was a really good and respected pupil, friend and colleague and will be sadly missed, though his effect will be lasting.

(Everton education welfare officer Mike Dickinson)

I can remember many, many times coming back on the team coach with Stockport from an away game, it would be 1am or 2am and Gary would be sat there still eager to talk about football. 'How do you think he did?' 'What about their winger?' That was Gary: always looking to learn, always looking to improve.

We had worked alongside each other at Liverpool, when Gary was reserve-team coach, and then at Stockport and our friendship and relationship grew stronger.

He was an excellent coach, who I have no doubt was going to make a name for himself in management, someone who led by example, who gave 100 per cent in everything he did and was always there for other people. Gary was a football man, but he was a fantastic person as well.

(Former Liverpool reserve and Stockport County coach Hughie McAuley)

He was a fantastic person, in the sense of being incredibly hard-working and incredibly positive at all times. He was a credit to himself and his family and to our football club during the time he worked with us. He had a big impact into the development of some of the young players while he was with us.

It is a very subdued place this morning (after news of Gary's death). It's our first day back and the normal routine would be wishing everyone a happy new year, so it's obviously very difficult this morning.

(Everton Academy coach Neil Dewsnip)

When Gary first crossed the park to Everton in 1992 I was a little wary – as most players probably are – of someone who has played for their fiercest rivals. When 'Abbo' left Everton FC in 1996, however, I thought of him as a friend, a top bloke and a lovely, lovely man.

He was the kind of fella you'd call if you fancied a pint – and you can't always say that about your team-mates. But such was Gary's personality and the way he conducted himself that he quickly became very popular at Goodison.

It takes a special kind of person to have the courage to make that move from Liverpool to Everton. Gary was under a lot of pressure when he made the switch, from fans of both sides, but the way he played and the way he conducted himself meant he won them all over.

He won the lads over at Everton. He mixed in straight away, but the only way you can win the respect of fellow professionals is if you can play, and Gary was an excellent footballer. You don't make as many appearances as he did for Liverpool without having quality.

He could play full-back or centre-back equally well because he was so comfortable in possession of the ball. But much more important than any football qualities he might have had, he was also a lovely lad.

I feel for his family and friends to lose someone at such a young age. And I think the reaction on both sides of Stanley Park will underline what a special person he was.

But I think the fact both sets of fans will mourn his passing equally is the biggest tribute to you can pay to him. Gary was a winner – for Liverpool and Everton – and he was also a top fella. Abbo, RIP.

(Everton team-mate Ian Snodin)

Gary was revered by both Reds and Blues, and that speaks volumes about the kind of player – and man – he was. We knew Gary had been seriously ill, but the news of his death is still very tough to take.

From a football point of view, Gary was under-rated. His team-mates didn't take him for granted as we knew how good he was but he didn't get the wider credit he deserved. He was a solid defender – not much got past him. He played in a tremendous Liverpool side in the late '80s.

He played a lot at left-back but could do a solid job anywhere along the back four. I remember him wearing that stupid hat after we had won the FA Cup in 1989. We had some great times.

In 1992 he was sold to Everton and he did a great job, helping them win the FA Cup a few years later. No-one had a bad word to say about Gary and he never let anyone down.

Gary was a great servant to both football clubs in the city. His death is a sad loss not only for Liverpool and Everton but for football. He was a talented coach and still had so much to offer. Rest in peace Gary.

(Liverpool team-mate John Aldridge)

Career Stats

First-team appearances – England only
(in chronological order – figures in
brackets represent goals)

Season	Club	Lge	FAC	LC	Eur	Other	Total
1984/85	Derby County (loan)	6	0	0	0	2	8
1985/86	Liverpool	0	0	0	0	0	0
1986/87	Hull City (loan)	5	0	0	0	0	5
	Liverpool	5 (1)	1	0	0	0	6 (1)
1987/88	Liverpool	17	5	0	0	0	22
1988/89	Liverpool	35	6	6	0	2	49
1989/90	Liverpool	15	0	1	0	0	16
1990/91	Liverpool	23	6	1	0	1	31
1991/92	Liverpool	14	0	3	6	0	23

Key:
FAC – FA Cup; LC – League Cup; Other – Includes Freight Rover Trophy (Hull City), FA Charity Shield (Liverpool and Everton), Football League Centenary Tournament (Liverpool), Auto Windscreens Shield (Blackpool)

CAREER STATS

First-team appearances (in England only)
(in chronological order – figures in brackets represent goals)

Season	Club	Lge	FAC	LC	Eur	Other	Total
1991/92	Everton	17 (1)	1	0	0	0	18 (1)
1992/93	Everton	40	2	6	0	0	48
1993/94	Everton	32 (1)	2	5	0	0	39 (1)
1994/95	Everton	26 (3)	4	0	0	0	30 (3)
1995/96	Everton	13	3 (1)	1	3	1	21 (1)
	Sheffield Utd (loan)	12	0	0	0	0	12
1996/97	Birmingham City	42 (1)	3	4	0	0	49 (1)
1997/98	Birmingham City	36	3 (1)	5	0	0	44 (1)
1998/99	Birmingham City	26	1	4	0	0	31
1999/00	Birmingham City	0	0	0	0	0	0
	Wycombe W. (loan)	4	0	0	0	0	4
	Blackpool	10 (1)	0	0	0	2	12 (1)

Key:
FAC – FA Cup; LC – League Cup; Other – Includes Freight Rover Trophy (Hull City), FA Charity Shield (Liverpool and Everton), Football League Centenary Tournament (Liverpool), Auto Windscreens Shield (Blackpool)

CLUB TOTALS

Club	Lge	FAC	LC	Eur	Other	Total
Derby County (loan)	6	0	0	0	2	8
Liverpool	109 (1)	18	11	6	3	147 (1)
Hull City (loan)	5	0	0	0	0	5
Everton	128 (5)	12 (1)	12	3	1	156 (6)
Sheffield United (loan)	12	0	0	0	0	12
Birmingham City	104 (1)	7 (1)	13	0	0	124 (2)
Wycombe Wan. (loan)	4	0	0	0	0	4
Blackpool	10 (1)	0	0	0	2	12 (1)
TOTAL	378 (8)	37 (2)	36	0	8	468 (10)

30th January 1985

Makes his professional debut as a 19-year-old, on loan at Derby County, in a 3-2 defeat by Bournemouth.

20th December 1986

Makes his Liverpool debut in a 0-0 draw with Charlton Athletic.

18th April 1987

Scores his only Liverpool goal on his home debut in a 3-0 win over Nottingham Forest – his 68th-minute strike completed the scoring.

23rd April 1988

Plays in the 1-0 victory over Tottenham Hotspur which confirmed Liverpool's 17th league title. His 17 league appearances for the 1987/88 campaign ensure a championship winner's medal.

14th May 1988

Starts in the 1988 FA Cup final defeat to Wimbledon at Wembley Stadium, having started every game from the fourth round onwards.

20th August 1988

A semblance of revenge is gained in the FA Charity Shield against Wimbledon, a 2-1 victory, with Gary again starting at Wembley.

1988/89 Season

Plays in 35 of Liverpool's 38 league games. He appears in 49 games in all – his best season for the Reds in terms of appearances.

20th May 1989

Won his first FA Cup winner's medal as Liverpool defeat Everton 3-2 after extra time.

CAREER STATS

1989/90 Season

Makes 15 appearances in the Reds' last title-winning season.

18th August 1990

Plays in the 1-1 FA Charity Shield draw with Manchester United.

1st January 1992

Makes the last of his 147 Liverpool appearances in a 2-1 league win over Sheffield United at Anfield.

11th January 1992

Agrees to join Everton for a fee of £750,000.

19th January 1992

Makes Blues debut in a 1-1 draw with Nottingham Forest.

29th February 1992

Scores his first Everton goal – and first for nearly five years – in a 2-0 away win at West Ham United.

7th May 1994

Survives the setback of a first-half own goal to help Everton defeat Wimbledon 3-2 to retain their top-flight status.

20th May 1995

Plays in the FA Cup final win over Manchester United and in doing so, becomes the only player to win the trophy with Liverpool and Everton; the first man to appear for Liverpool and Everton in Wembley FA Cup finals; the only player to appear for and against Everton in an FA Cup final; and one of only two players to have won an FA Cup winner's medal with Liverpool and another club – Ray Clemence is the other.

13th August 1995

Plays in the FA Charity Shield, with Everton defeating Premier League champions Blackburn Rovers 1-0 at Wembley.

Summer 1996

After helping Sheffield United stay up in Division One, joins Birmingham City for £390,000. He makes his Blues debut on 18th August, a 1-0 home victory over Crystal Palace.

14th February 1998

Scores his second – and final – goal for Birmingham City in a 3-2 FA Cup fifth-round defeat at Premier League Leeds United. His previous strike had come in a defeat at Swindon Town the previous campaign.

6th February 1999

Picks up serious injury in the first half of a 1-1 draw at Crystal Palace. It proves to be his final appearance for Blues.

7th January 2000

Joins his final English club, Blackpool, on non-contract terms having spent most of December 1999 on loan with Wycombe Wanderers. He makes his debut four days later, a 1-0 victory at Mansfield Town in the Auto Windscreens Shield.

15th January 2000

Nets the 10th and final goal of his career, for Blackpool, in a 3-3 draw with Luton Town.

11th March 2000

Makes his 468th and final career appearance as a first-half substitute in a 2-2 draw against Cardiff City at Bloomfield Road.

Index